YOUR NORTHEAST BACKYARD HOMESTEAD

WHAT TO PLANT, HOW TO PLANT, AND WHEN TO PLANT FOR YOUR CLIMATE

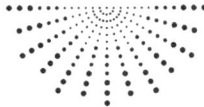

J. B. MAXWELL

For my son, may the world be your garden and may you grow whatever you choose to.

CONTENTS

Introduction   9

1. KNOW YOUR CLIMATE   17
   Climate in the Northeast   20

2. THE LAY OF THE LAND   23

3. BUILDING YOUR BEDS   31
   Strategies for Making the Most of Your
   Raised Beds   34

4. HOMESTEADING FOR THE WIN   41
   Getting Settled   47
   Raising Animals   54
   Composting   63
   Ideal Plant Environments   66
   Maximizing Your Yield   77

5. ESSENTIAL SOIL   83

6. INCORPORATING PERMACULTURE   93
   Ethics and Principles of Permaculture
   Design   95
   Perennial and Annual Plants   105

7. SPRING   107
   Spring Vegetables   109
   Spring Fruits and Herbs   113
   Spring Flowers   115

8. SUMMER   121
   Summer Vegetables   122
   Summer Fruits and Herbs   124
   Summer Flowers   127

9. FALL   131
   Fall Vegetables   133
   Fall Fruits and Herbs   136
   Fall Flowers   139

10. WINTER   141
   Winter Trees and Shrubs   144

11. TIPS AND TRICKS FOR ULTIMATE
   SUCCESS   149
   Optimizing the Space on Your
   Property   152
   Planting Success   153
   Insect Management   156

   Afterword   161
   References   167

indirect, that are incurred as a result of the use of the information contained within this document, including, but not limited to, errors, omissions, or inaccuracies.

❀ Created with Vellum

INTRODUCTION

Let the beauty you love be what you do
— RUMI

It is possible that you are feeling run down and burned out from living in an urban environment. You could want to cut down on living expenses and get back in touch with nature, or you could be someone who is driven by self-sustainable practices. No matter the case, living off the grid or partially off the grid can help you find solutions to a lot of the stress and turmoil of everyday life. This book is a guide for how to start a new off-the-grid property in the Northeast and make the most of homesteading practices. I will go through the initial phases on your property, how to best plan your success, and the needs that your Northeast farm will have during each of the four seasons.

Living in the Northeast means that you will constantly be surrounded by beautiful landscapes and experience all that the four seasons have to offer. However, while the Northeast can be beautiful, starting a homestead in the Northeast can come with its own challenges, especially if you are looking to live off the grid. Northeast farmers face drastic temperature changes that they must account for when they are developing a garden, and a wide range of pests and insects that will be attracted to their gardens. The freezing temperatures that parts of the Northeast experience for large portions of the year also add to the challenges of starting a farm. Nevertheless, starting a homestead in the Northeast is an incredibly fulfilling process that requires time, attention to detail, and labor. By the end of your first or second year on your property you will have bountiful harvests and a gorgeous farm that will make all the effort of living in the Northeast worth it.

According to the Conservation Institute, over 1.7 billion people are living off the grid, meaning they do not rely on public utilities for electricity and water. In addition to that, over 250,000 people in the United States live off the grid and over 1.7 billion people around the globe live off the grid. In 2019, 79 million households used solar energy to fuel their off the grid homes (BigRentz, 2020). The benefits of living off the grid are clearly driving more and more people to cut the cord. Some of these benefits are self-sufficiency, a better connection with nature, improvements in conserving energy, and a generally more environmentally friendly life. Living off the grid can considerably cut down the costs of living in an average home. Most people in the United States spend over $2,000 a year on utility bills (BigRentz, 2020). In 2017, the energy consumption for a four family house in the United States was 10,399 kWh. While this may seem fine, reducing your energy intake can improve your carbon footprint. Right now, in the United States, renewable energy only accounts for 11% of energy consumption while the rest is used for fossil fuels (BigRentz, 2020). I don't expect that you are drilling for oil or that you are solely responsible for fossil fuel energy consumption, but to offset the impacts of climate change as a result of fossil fuels, improving your renewable energy consumption can help.

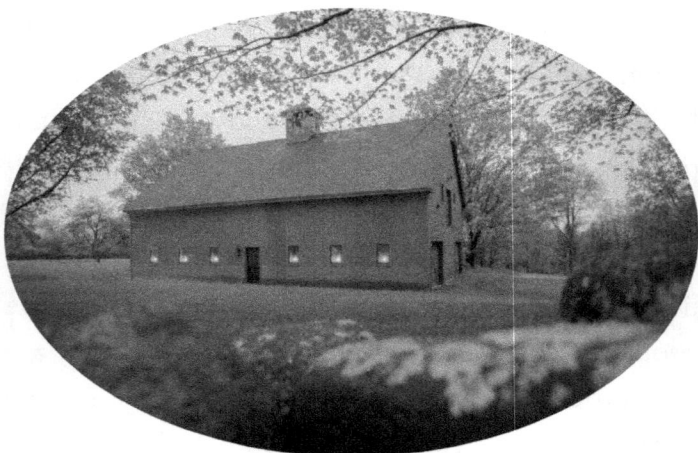

Living off the grid can also mean drastically reducing your costs of living. If you don't have rent and utilities to pay for, you will have more capital to invest toward your farm and property. The following figures for off-the-grid farming are subject to changes based on the location and time that you are looking to develop a homestead. Some of the initial costs to living off the grid include the cost of land, electricity, heating, water, waste management, and food. Finding the right land for your homestead is highly dependent on where in the world you want to be. In the United States and Canada, 5 acres of land typically costs about $3,000 per acre. You will want to save about $15,000 if you are considering buying a property with no existing structures on it.

There are many options when considering how you will power your house. A lot of off-the-grid homesteaders will opt for solar energy. Solar panels range in price and quality; the average cost per watt for solar panels is about $3. If you have a 2,500-square-foot home, you will need to save about $20,000 for solar panels. In addition, many states offer tax incentives and other benefits if you opt into sustainable energy for your property. The alternative options are wind power and hydro power to power your home, which also range in cost. You will want to consider what the most abundant source for renewable power is on your property. If you have a large pond or river, investing in a hydropower system may be more prudent.

Similar to power, heating your home can also have a lot of options. Geothermal heat pumps, solar heating, and biomass boiler systems are all possible considerations. Again, for a 2,500-square-foot home, you will want to save about $7,500 for a heating system. A water pump, well, or rainwater collection system are all options for considering how you will get clean water into your off-the-grid home. I highly recommend that if you are starting your first property, you buy a plot of land that already has a well on it. It can be very costly to dig a new well: depending on how deep you will need to dig for water, and the type of system you choose to have, you will want to save about $6,000 to $10,000 for a water system. Waste management is probably the most controversial area that you will need to consider for off-the-grid living. A septic tank or composting toilet are both options for waste management. Septic tanks require a lot of money upfront to have installed. I would estimate saving another $6,000 for a waste management system. These prices will vary a lot depending on if you are building structures yourself, updating existing structures, or paying a contractor to build these structures on your property.

Finding food for yourself and your family is where the homesteading aspect of living off the grid begins. There are many prudent methods for establishing your homestead so that you have access to high-quality foods that cost a fraction of the price that they would in a grocery store. Depending on the size of your property and the space that you want to allot to crops, gardening, and raising livestock, I would recommend saving about $30,000 to $35,000 for your off-the-grid farm. In total, starting such a homestead will run about $80,000 to $90,000 at the outset. The benefit of this initial investment is that beyond the maintenance that you will have to do on your property, additional costs will be incredibly low (BigRentz, 2020).

I have been homesteading for 10 years and during my time I have made many mistakes trying to figure out the best way to run my farm. Now, I want to offer you some sage advice about how you can thrive on your new property. Even if you haven't made the purchase yet, *Your Northeast Backyard Homestead* can help you put into perspective the benefits of living in nature and being self-sustaining.

1

KNOW YOUR CLIMATE

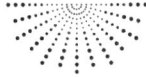

*H*omesteading is an incredibly beneficial process that you can engage with if you are someone who prioritizes working in nature, self-sustainability, and self-reliance. In the Northeast, homesteading can be slightly trickier because of the climate. In this geographical area there are drastic seasonal changes that require an extra level of preparedness when you are planning your property: cold winters, short and at times humid summers, early frost, just to name a few.

However, before I begin talking about the specifics that are required when you are starting a homestead in the Northeast, it is important to cover what exactly homesteading is. Homesteading is the practice of living a self-sufficient and -sustainable lifestyle. Many styles of homesteading call for off-the-grid living and self-reliance, but it is possible to create an urban or apartment homestead as well to begin practicing different methods before you even invest in this lifestyle. The Homestead Act of 1862 was the act that stated that any public land in the western regions of the United States could be granted to any citizen to farm on for 5 years. Similarly in Canada, there was an act in 1872 called the Dominion Lands Act that espoused a similar standard. Both of these acts were put in place to encourage more people to move out of urban areas and foster agricultural industries. In the continental United States, nearly 10% of all the land was allotted to homesteaders as a result of the act (Culver, 2021).

Homesteading today has taken on many different forms. There are options for both urban and rural families to practice different homesteading techniques to become more self-sustaining. If you are living in an urban or suburban area and you are interested in a more self-sustaining life, try starting small. Beginning with a small garden on your balcony, collecting rainwater, or cultivating yeast are great small steps to take when starting your journey with homesteading. Another great option is to get your family engaged. A backyard garden, small chicken coop, or a rabbit coop are great for smaller children to engage with. There are essential life lessons that children can glean from hard work and a sense of fulfillment when they see their first crop blossom. Needless to say, homesteading is a way to sustain yourself and find a greater sense of self-reliance. The cost of living, the bustle of urban life, and a dependency on your own work will all provide a mindset for homesteading that is pivotal to the process.

One of the benefits of starting a homestead in the Northeast is the weather changes and varied pursuits that you can start on your property. You can do anything, from building a greenhouse, planting a typical garden or crop field, to raising animals, and many other ventures. The region in the United States that is called the Northeast spans from the southernmost point of New Jersey and goes up through the northernmost points in Maine. If you are considering living in the Northeast in the United States, it is important to note that global temperatures are slightly rising and the Northeast has seen a lot of climate changes as a result. The average summer temperatures have risen by 2 °F over the last 100 years, and as a result there have been longer summer heat waves, an increase in rainfall, and slightly shorter winter seasons in the northern parts of this region (US EPA, 2016). Where I live in Pennsylvania, we see temperatures as high as 95 °F in the summer time to 10 °F in the winter. These temperature changes absolutely impact what and when I choose to plant in my gardens. I keep a calendar where I track the first and last frosts of the year to give me insight on when I should start planting outdoors and when I should start seeds in my greenhouse. While these dates change from year to year, I have found that keeping an eye on the forecast and planning accordingly has helped my garden thrive.

CLIMATE IN THE NORTHEAST

Approximately, 64 million people live in the Northeast of the United States. With more than 180,000 farms that annually net $17 billion, the Northeast is a great place to start your homesteading journey (National Climate Assessment, 2021). The landscape in the Northeast is largely made up of forests. There are some grasslands, beaches, and wetlands. There is also a large fishing industry. The region is characterized by a diverse climate that sees about 20 inches of rain per year, depending on the proximity to the coast and elevation. The area also sees floods, heat waves, hurricanes, and nor'easters (big snowstorms!). There is always a chance that living in the Northeast will mean that you will have to invest in a backup generator as a result of some of the weather patterns in the region. In 2016, we got nearly 20 inches of snow in January, which led to power outages across my state. On my property, I had a backup generator, survival storage, and a lot of candles stocked up in case we lost power. I knew that buying a property in the Northeast meant that power outages could be a possibility, and I was so happy that we had planned for the inevitability of one. We were living comfortably while the snow came down outside, or at least I was until it came time to start shoveling the snow.

The average temperatures in the Northeast during the year range from 26 °F to 85 °F, and in some areas the winter temperatures can fall below 14 °F and the summers can see temperatures above 93 °F. According to WeatherSpark, the Northeast is one of the most extreme regions in the United States that sees humidity variation throughout the year. The humid season in the Northeast lasts from the end of May until the end of September. The most humid month of the year is July, with an average of

19 days that will reach 66% humidity. The clearest months in the Northeast are from the end of June until the first weeks of November. The clearest month in the Northeast is September. The cloudiest parts of the year in the Northeast last from November until the middle of June. The cloudiest month during the year in the Northeast is January, with 52% of the sky covered in clouds throughout the month (WeatherSpark, 2020). The rain season in the Northeast lasts from the beginning of April until the end of August; the rainiest month of the year is July, with an average of 11 rain days per month. The inverse of the rainy season is the drier season of the year, with January being the month that sees the least amount of precipitation. Precipitation in the Northeast accounts for both the rain and snow seasons.

2

THE LAY OF THE LAND

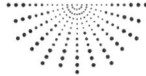

When you are thinking about the size of your property and what will be the best amount of land to fit your needs, I would recommend considering your budget. There are so many options for property sizes, depending on where in the Northeast you are looking to settle down. I remember when I bought my first plot of land. It was 1 acre, and yet I felt out of my element when it came to filling up the space and utilizing it in the best way possible. When you are starting this journey, consider what you will want to spend your time doing and the space that can accommodate those activities. I personally love having a small garden near my kitchen, raising some small furry friends, and leaving space for my family to enjoy nature.

A great first step is to consider the goals that you have for your property. Consider your answers to the following questions:

- How much time do you expect (or want) to spend maintaining your property?
- How much time do you want to spend outdoors enjoying nature, not working?
- How much land do you have available to dedicate to gardening or raising animals?
- What are the local ordinances in your area?
- Do you want to turn homesteading into your full-time job?
- How involved will your family be in your homesteading journey?

These questions may be tricky to answer at first if you are still narrowing down your property options. Once you have your sights set on a piece of land, consider your answers to these questions and remember, it is perfectly acceptable if the answers change over time. The next step that I encourage all beginners to take is to create a list of your homesteading goals, the amount of land that you will need to dedicate to those goals, and the materials that you will need on hand to build and maintain that area. For example, if you want to keep a small kitchen garden outside of your backdoor, you will probably want to allot about 0.1 acre to that area. For livestock, you will want to have 1 to 3 acres of space, depending on the animals. Keep in mind that smaller animals need less room than larger livestock. Each goal that you list for your property will require certain tools to build the structures and maintain the systems you put in place. When I started my first homestead, I was convinced that I wanted to raise some rabbits. I built a handful of hutches for them, but during certain seasons it was difficult to get my hands on the right hay for their enclosures. I didn't make a list of the resources that I would need to maintain the area, so I came up against an avoidable hurdle. You don't have to be like me in the beginning! My goal is that you can learn some of the strategies that I have developed so that you can avoid those mishaps.

After you have established your goals, I recommend that you spend some time thinking about how self-sustaining you want to be. If your goal is to go totally off the grid, you will probably require more land than someone who is staying on the grid and still buying food from the grocery store. I am by no means saying that one method is more legitimate than the other, but if you are going for the off-the-grid method, it is always better to consider getting a larger piece of land. However, with strategic planning and consideration of your goals, you don't actually need that much space to start a homestead. A lot of processes can be rotated out of areas on your property so that you are making the most of the land!

There are endless creative options to pursue when you are starting your first homestead. In the Northeast, there is a lot of available land, but if you need to ask yourself: What is the smallest amount of land that I could have to start a traditional farm? The minimum amount of land that you can have for a homestead is about an acre. Keep in mind that with an acre of land, you will probably only be able to have a garden. For animals or a forest to harvest wood, you will need 2 to 10 acres. This is not to say that this is the only way to start a farm. There are a lot of urban homesteading options where people have developed creative solutions to limited space. I have a friend who lives in Boston who works on a cooperative farming operation out of shipping containers. They utilize vertical farming and aquaponic farming to achieve the same results that someone would achieve on a large rural farm. When you center self-sustainability in your practice of farming, the options for how to make accommodations for your space are endless. However, this book will focus on the starter farm that will range from 1 acre to about 5 acres.

Now that you have an understanding of the space required to farm, your goals for your property, and the mindset that is essential when you are starting this journey, it is time to consider the nuances of your property. For a small garden the essential components of laying out your area are the accessibility, light, safety, and plant health. When you are considering the accessibility of your property, it is crucial to think about how far away aspects of your farm are. It is a great practice to consider permaculture zones to inform the layout of your farm. The general rule is that you want to keep things closer to the house on your property that will need daily attention. I will discuss more of the details of permaculture design in Chapter 6.

Once you have decided where you will place your garden and the first structures on your property, consider the light and safety that your plants will need. Access to sunlight, shade, and a lack of wind will be pivotal to a successful garden. In the Northeast, there are many months in the year where your plants will get direct sunlight. Depending on the crops that you want to grow, they will need different access to sunlight. Consider a space on your property that gets both direct sunlight and shade so that your plants can thrive. Keep in mind that if the garden is too close to your house, the garden will be shaded considerably by the shadow cast by the house. Be careful in the planning phase to think about the direction of the sun throughout the entire day and at different times of the year. The general rule is to keep your garden at least 10 feet away from any walls of your house. You will also want to see how much wind your area gets. In the Northeast, there are seasons that are windier than others. This step can be completed before you move onto your property. Regional maps of your area can indicate the average wind speeds that your farm will experience. Consider if the wind speeds on the property will be too rough during some months of the year and how that can damage your crops. Typically, crops don't love an excess of wind: their leaves can be damaged or the entire plant could be uprooted, leading to a headache and a mess. While this may seem like a minor setback, if you are staking your meals and income on the success of your plants, be sure that you research and observe your farm so that you can have a thriving garden.

With the age of technology, finding all of the information about a plot of land you are interested in purchasing before you buy has become incredibly accessible. I regularly hop on Google and look for properties that I find interesting. As an exercise, I will plot out the best farming layout for the property to see if I can catch every contingency that needs to be thought through. Google Maps is a great resource in this process because you can get a fairly detailed look at the property from an aerial view. When it comes time to actually choose a property, there are some other calls that you can make to get even more information about the area. Contacting the local utility companies is a great practice because there may be wiring or pipes under your property and it would be a mess if you accidentally dug into one. All of the Northeast states have Dig Safe laws that require you to notify the county if you are going to be excavating on your property in order to go about the process safely. Failing to adhere to the Dig Safe laws in your area can result in hefty fines. Calling utility companies or contacting your county to learn about your property and what might be hiding underneath your property can give you great insights on where to plan different aspects of your farm. It may be the case that you have a city water pipe under your property that prohibits you from farming over it. This is a great way to narrow down the options you have for where to place your gardens.

3

BUILDING YOUR BEDS

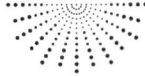

*W*hen you are planning the best ways to grow crops in your garden, raised beds are a great option that maximize harvests and protect your plants. Raised beds are garden beds that are built above the ground instead of into the ground. There are many different methods for how to achieve a raised garden bed. Often you will see wood panels or larger steel drums that enclose the raised bed. Raised beds are also sometimes referred to as 'garden boxes.' The purpose of gardening above the ground instead of directly into the soil is that you can better control the pH of the soil, the depth of the roots, and protect your crops from pests that may damage your plants.

In addition, some benefits of using raised beds on

your farm are improved soil quality, improved soil drainage, ease of gardening, longer growing seasons, and cultivating an aesthetic form. Not tilling the soil is better for your plants. When you are setting up your raised beds or maintaining them between seasons, you will be able to add fertilizer, soil, and compost to the top of the bed without the added work of tilling the ground. This creates a faster process, where you have more control over the nutrients and soil quality that your plants are getting. Raised beds also keep pests out of your garden more effectively than planting directly into the ground. Many of the garden pests that you will want to protect your plants from cannot climb up the sides of the raised bed and will be discouraged from trying to eat your crops. Similarly, in the Northeast, there is a large deer population that will definitely be attracted to your crops. With a raised bed, it is easier to add deer fencing above the crops so that the deers cannot access the leafy green vegetables that they love. When I set up my first raised bed, I wanted to plant some strawberries, borage, and mint into my raised beds. The borage and mint are deer favorites and I knew that spending a little extra time to secure my raised beds would mean that I got a great harvest at the end of the season that was not littered with deer bites. I also opted to plant some shrubs on the edges of my property so that the deers could have a snack that I was less invested in if they happened to stop by.

Raised beds also offer better soil drainage. One of the trickiest pieces of setting up a homestead is your water supply and drainage. It takes a lot of careful consideration to set up the water system on your farm so that you are not overwatering your crops or underutilizing the water at your disposal. With raised beds, because of their height, the soil is able to drain quicker and keep your plants healthier longer. The standard raised bed is between 11 and 12 inches high. This is the perfect height that plants need for drainage. If you are living in an area that is prone to flooding, which is common in some areas of the Northeast, raised beds may be your only option for high-quality farming. Otherwise you will run the risk of your plants drowning or being overwatered. Similarly, if you are in an area that gets a lot of rain, the 12-inch raised beds will allow the soil to drain at a consistent rate without risking the health of your crops. An additional benefit to raised beds is that they can elevate some of the back-breaking work that gardening calls for. With the beds being raised off the ground, you can avoid spending hours hunched over tending to your garden. The beds also make weeding much easier.

Good soil drainage in your raised beds is great if you are using raised beds to feed your family or community. The crops will be fresh and delicious, as well as abundant. Keep in mind, this largely works because of soil quality and density. You will want to ensure that your soil is the correct pH and you are adding the proper nutrients so that your plants can thrive. The last benefit of raised beds is that they are really pretty. Your garden will look neat and contained. You can easily plant crops in a single raised bed that compliment one another. Your garden will undoubtedly look lush and vibrant if you utilize raised beds on your farm.

STRATEGIES FOR MAKING THE MOST OF YOUR RAISED BEDS

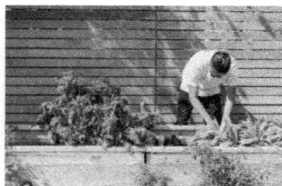

So how do you actually go about building raised beds? There are many different methods for building them and the materials that you use can vary. The general rule to building raised beds with wooden sides is that you avoid using pressure-treated wood. Plywood and other chemically treated woods can leach chemicals into your soil and compromise your plants' health. If you have never built a raised bed before but you are interested in having some on your farm, Home Depot offers raised garden bed plans and kits that will make your life easier as you start your farming journey. If you have a little more experience with building and want to cut down on cost, a great method for building a raised bed is to buy cedar planks the length, width, and height of your raised bed, as well as 2 × 2 or 4 × 4 pieces of wood for the corners of your raised bed. The cedar planks can be any size that works for your farm as long as you get four planks to surround the area that you are building your raised bed in. I highly suggest that the height of your raised beds be 12 inches so that you get the best soil drainage as possible. The corner pieces should be taller than the height of your raised bed so that you can secure netting or other protective measures over the top of the bed.

Another strategy that a lot of raised bed gardeners use is called 'lasagna gardening.' This is the process of layering multiple layers of mulch, compost, and other organic materials into your raised bed to improve the soil quality and nutrients that your plants receive. There is no standard for how to lasagna garden, but in my experience, I have had the most success when I have layered branches and rough mulch over the ground, then grass clippings, wet newspaper, compost, and straw mulch. Be sure that you water each layer as you place them into your garden. This is also a great way to cut down on cost as you will be able to find most of the materials for lasagna gardening on your farm already. Of course, you can always add the soil of your choice for specific crops if you want to ensure that they get the exact pH or nutrients that are required for them to grow.

Some alternative raised garden bed methods are fabric raised planters, elevated raised gardens that usually require adding legs to your garden box, tiered raised beds, galvanized metal raised beds, trough raised beds, and many others. The benefit of raised beds is that you can be endlessly creative in the materials used to contain the small gardens. I have even seen people make their raised beds in old tires! The possibilities are endless and you can utilize the materials that you have available to you on your farm or you can invest in store-bought materials to create the gardens.

Now that you know why people use raised beds,

the benefits of the small gardens, and some additional design ideas for how to build the beds, there are some things that you will need to prepare before you start building. You will first want to identify the space on your farm that is ideal for the garden. Remember, you want to have your gardens relatively close to your house so that you can monitor them regularly, but not so close that the gardens are prone to shadow for too many hours a day. Another consideration to make is if you want to remove the grass from below the raised beds. Some farmers will take the time to cut out the grass patches below so that they can plant deeper into the raised beds. This isn't an entirely necessary process if you aren't planting deep-rooting crops. However, if you decide to remove the grass from under your raised beds, a great strategy that will cut down on time is to place the raised beds on your farm at the end of the fall season: place a layer of cardboard or newspaper over the ground and let the grass decay over the winter. At the start of the spring, you will have a grassless area.

Irrigation is another consideration that you will need to make before you finish the construction of your garden. Raised beds that are made out of galvanized steel or trough call for irrigation systems that are a little more intense and require a water hookup for them to be successful. For the traditional raised bed, you can add a pipe that runs through the bottom third, with holes in it. The pipe can be connected to a rain collection bin or a water pump and you can automate the watering process. Otherwise, it is perfectly acceptable to add 'watering your crops' to your list of daily farm chores!

Here are some additional tips and tricks to consider when you are starting your garden of raised beds:

- The first crops that you start planting in your raised garden beds should be the herbs and vegetables that you will want to eat. Herbs are very forgiving crops that can withstand a little neglect. Developing your own systems to tend to the crops that you will most enjoy will make the gardening experience all the more fulfilling.
- If you have any areas where you raised beds are more shaded, plant leafy greens. Most crops will benefit from 6 to 8 hours of sunlight per day, but leafy greens can handle a little less sunlight and still thrive.

Plant spinach, borage, and lettuce in the more shaded areas of your garden.

- Keep a ledger of the crops that you plant from year to year. Having a way to track the crops that were planted in a specific raised bed will inform you on what to plant the following year and the accommodations that you will need to make to the soil, compost, and mulch that is still in the raised bed.

- Along with keeping a ledger of your crops, when you go to plant your seedlings, be sure that you are planting them in rows. This will ensure that the weeding and tending processes are faster and easier. Also, planting your crops in rows will mean that you don't accidentally pull up one of your crops because you mistakenly thought it was a weed (and believe me, weeds are masters at impersonation).

- Consider companion planting when you are planning your raised beds. I will dig deeper into the benefits of companion planting in Chapter 4, but when you are considering what to plant, some crops get along nicely with others and can be planted in the same bed. Companion planting will also maximize your harvests as the crops have a symbiotic relationship with each other.

- Plant annual cover crops like ryegrass or clover. These cover crops can be seeded into your raised beds at the start of spring and will provide necessary nitrogen and other nutrients to your raised beds between growing seasons. Plus, a bunch of clover peeking out from your raised beds during the non-growing seasons is really adorable.

4

HOMESTEADING FOR THE WIN

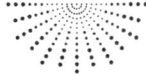

*T*here are a couple more steps to cover before you actually get on to your new property. When you first start this process, it is not only important to plan systems for your success but also to ensure that you have a mindset that will lend itself to a prosperous adventure. One of the most key aspects to tackling a new property or a brand new journey is to push yourself to continue to learn. There are thousands of resources available to you on your homesteading journey that can inform your practices and projects on your farm. It is vital that you find creative solutions to different systems on your property and continue to innovate. While there are a lot of steps to the planning phase of your journey, once you start implementing systems it is important to continue to learn about those systems. You may have a well on your property that you are using to water your gardens and provide water to your home, but what happens in the winter if the water in the well freezes? Finding creative solutions and learning more about systems like water distribution will be prudent to making a homestead last. The mentality to continue to learn is essential to setting up your property for longevity and success.

Now that you are driven to continue to learn, it is important to be able to think critically about how the information that you have gathered fits your situation. While I encourage everyone to dig into the resources at your disposal, they will not be useful to you if you can't apply them to your situation. I remember reading about keeping bees on my homestead and I was really excited to start a beekeeping project on my farm. However, when I got to the property, I realized that I would have to do a lot of work upfront to prepare for the bees. I needed to clear some space, plant pollinating flowers near where I wanted to place the beehives, and get the equipment necessary to keep bees. While the information that I got was vital, it would have been useless if I didn't apply my own situation to the information. Applying the information that you are getting from other resources to your situation can help you avoid unnecessary time loss while you are navigating how the project will work for you.

In addition, it may be tempting to get all of the information about different projects for your homestead from online resources, but I want to encourage you to get help and information from other sources as well. There are vibrant communities both online and in person that you can participate in when you are discovering new information or when you come up against a hurdle. Asking for help when you need it from trusted sources is another mindset shift that every new property owner needs in order to be successful. I will talk at more length about the benefits of cultivating relationships with your neighbors in a later part of this chapter, but for now, the importance of joining or cultivating relationships with trusted people is paramount. If you find that you are in a bind and need help, the internet may provide you with information that is general but it won't fit directly to your situation. If you have the ability to explain your exact situation to a trusted friend or neighbor, or even the owner of the local gardening nursery or hardware store, you will receive much more sage advice on how to proceed.

The next mindset that every farmer should have

is to be aware of how much you can take on. Be honest with yourself while you are planning the projects that you want to have on your farm. How much can you reasonably do in a day and how much effort do you want to put into different projects? Maybe you want to only spend your time gardening. How many hours of the day can you do that? What if you only want to raise rabbits and maintain a small kitchen garden on the side? Discover exactly how much time and effort you want to put into different projects and then budget at least half the amount of time to unexpected situations. In the Northeast, there are bound to be weather events or storms that will throw your perfect systems into disarray. You can have some animals on your farm that get sick and you will need to spend extra time caring for them. Or you may not have protected your coops enough and your animals get targeted by predators. There are always going to be unexpected twists and turns, the goal is to accurately determine how much time you can spend doing the things that make you happy while budgeting time for those unexpected events. This will also ensure that you are not constantly exhausted from having to run around your farm all day because you planned to accomplish too many different tasks. I personally love to take a day off every week so that I can read and relax. When I first started my farm, I knew that I had to set up systems so that at least one day a week, I could take some time off for myself and my family.

Once you have established some ideas for what you want on your farm and how much time and energy you can devote to those things, it is time to consider your finances. Making smart financial decisions that won't ultimately be detrimental to your success is a tricky process, but it is one that every farmer needs to master. There are going to be financial investments that you will need to make into building materials, seeds, and animals, but all of those investments come with added costs. You may want to raise chickens and they will need a coop, pen, and feed. The profit that you make from selling the eggs or meat may not cover the initial costs that it took to raise them. It is important to consider all of the expenses for the projects that you want to start and the type of return on your investments that you can expect. In addition, you will want to consider the market that you are selling into. With the age of technology, there are many money-making practices that you can capitalize on while you are homesteading. However, if you take a more traditional route and sell your produce or animals locally, there may already be sellers in your area and the market for your goods might not be available.

Making these considerations before you get onto your property will ensure that you don't waste money on the initial investments to set up a project without turning a profit down the line. It's the same as writing a business plan for a new venture. I suggest setting up a list of the projects you want to accomplish, the cost of every aspect of those projects, and what types of profit you may be able to reap from those projects. For example, if you want to raise chickens, consider all of the costs involved in raising the chickens and the types of profit that you can make from them depending on your area. It is also especially important to consider the weather in addition to finances. What costs are associated with keeping your chickens warm during the winter or ensuring that their water bowls don't freeze? How will it impact your finances if a predator gets into the coop and wipes out the flock?

There are also areas that you can invest in that will yield higher profits than others. Your garden is a great example of this. The cost of seeds is very low and setting up your garden doesn't have to be a particularly costly venture. Selling your produce will net you a lot more than your initial investment. The goal is to find the right market to sell to. Regardless of the type of profits that you are expecting to reap from your farm, I want to warn you that the return on your money will probably be slower than you are expecting. For your first homestead, there are a lot of other considerations that need to be made and systems to put in place before turning a profit becomes a viable option. The last and arguably most important mindset that every new farmer needs to have is that homesteading is a long-term investment: you may invest years into a project before that project pays off the initial investment. The homesteading lifestyle transcends the money-making ventures that you could make and there are many benefits to being outside in nature and living a less fast-paced life. Keep in mind that while it will feel fulfilling to make money from your hard work, the real goal of homesteading is to spend time on your farm doing things that make you happy.

GETTING SETTLED

So what do you do when you have your property? The best piece of advice that I can give you is to start slowly. It could be argued that this is another mindset shift that you will need to engage with before you start your farm, but starting slow and ensuring that you are comfortable on your property before you start tackling larger projects will be key to your success in the first year on your property. When you get the keys to your property, don't do everything right away. It is important to feel settled before you can begin to tackle the different projects you want to start. I have heard a lot of stories of people getting to their homestead and immediately starting a garden, while all of their clothes and furniture were still in boxes. Feeling settled on your property will provide you more space and time to dedicate to fleshing out the projects that you want to accomplish and to do them in a well-thought out manner. There are also a lot of benefits to planning out the space in your home. Once you start tackling different tasks on your farm, you will need to set up systems inside your house that will promote those projects. You may be growing a lot of food, but how will you store the food? Do you want to can or pickle your harvests so that you can preserve them? You will need to have some extra cabinet or refrigerator space to keep your preserves fresh. Unpack your things and set up systems inside your house for success before you begin tackling bigger projects on your farm.

Another great first step to take once you get onto your property is to meet your neighbors. This is going to be especially crucial if you are living in a rural place. You may have less access to resources and developing solid relationships with your neighbors can lead to fostering a community where you help one another. In rural areas, it will take a lot more time to get certain resources and you will be responsible for the general maintenance of structures around you. It may be the case that you are sharing roads or fences with your neighbors and if they need repairs; it will be far easier to get those jobs done if you enjoy being around each other and are clear as to who owns what and who is responsible for those areas. Working cooperatively with the people in your community can be a saving grace on your first homestead. In addition to meeting your neighbors, it is important to understand the access issues that you may encounter on your property. Living in more rural places will require that you know everything about the land around you. If you are living in the Northeast, there is a large possibility that you will get snowed into your house. Knowing where the access roads are, having access to a snowplow, and relying on your neighbors will be crucial. It is also important to know where power lines and water pipes are. This will give you more insight into the area. You can get this information from your neighbors as well as the county.

Living in a state of preparedness will also be essential once you move into your new property. Storage and survival storage are really important systems to have set up early on when you move into your new home. Buy the food that you need in bulk and preserve it in areas that you've set up in your home. There may be busy days or emergencies that will require you to have extra food on hand: for example, if you have a day where cooking seems like too much effort because you're dealing with an emergency or you get snowed in. Another aspect of preparedness that is essential to consider is your access to water. It is very likely that your house will already have running water unless you are building your house on your own. I highly recommend buying a property that already has a well on it so that you can start gardening projects when you are ready. Otherwise, you will need to devise creative irrigation systems around your farm. Inside your house, be sure that you keep an extra tank of water on hand if you are in a relatively rural place so that there is no chance that you will run out of water if there is a power outage or some sort of weather intervention that would prevent you from accessing water.

Along the same lines as storing excess water, be sure that you also store excess power and fuel. Living in the Northeast comes with extreme weather events that may make getting electricity or fuel more difficult. Ensure that you have extra fuel containers to power your car or a backup generator. The way that you choose to power your house will also come into play as you first move in. For off-the-grid homes, there are many types of renewable energy sources that require initial investments to install. Regardless of your power source, it is always a great practice to keep a backup generator on hand in case of a storm. The last thing that you should have on hand in case of emergencies or distances from a hospital, are medical supplies. Be sure that you have first-aid kits and any extra medical supplies that you or your family will need on your property. Taking these necessary precautions and prioritizing preparedness when you start on your first homestead will make it so that you are ready for any situation.

Another step to take once you get the keys to your new property is to observe your land. I will discuss later the key aspects to permaculture design, which will provide you with insights on how to best lay out your farm projects. However, when you first get onto your property, observe how the existing structures on your farm will influence the layout of your property. Observe how different organic structures on your farm will impact the day-to-day experience on your farm. You may have a little dip in the land that floods when it rains. It would be hard to preemptively know that this would happen and you would hate to place a raised bed in that area, only for it to get destroyed or compromised when it rains. There are many other observations that you will make in the first couple of weeks on the homestead. These observations will inform how you begin planning the layout of your farm without accidentally placing a structure in an inopportune spot. After a couple of weeks of unpacking and observing your property, it is time to plan all of the zones on your farm before you start your projects. The general rules for permaculture design are that you want the areas that are closest to your home to be the areas that you visit and maintain regularly. The farther away you get from your home, the less those areas require maintenance. Observing your property first is imperative to discovering the best way to do this.

At this point you should have a general idea of

how you are going to plan out your farm and what projects you will want to start building. The next step is to *continue* planning, as there are going to be many different areas on your property that will require some detailed thought and preparation before you can start building or developing processes. Plan before you start gardening, plan before you start coppicing trees, and plan before you buy animals. How are you going to maintain your animals and where can they graze? Be sure that they have an area to roam outside of their enclosures. Think about the feed that they will need. Also consider how you are going to store all of the resources for your animals and how that storage process will be affected in the winter. Be sure that you secure a local veterinarian. This is also a moment where neighbors become great resources. If you have a neighbor who is also raising animals, they may know a local veterinarian who makes house calls or they may know how to identify or treat issues that your animals may be having, so you don't need to call the veterinarian every time (as vet bills can add up!). All of this is to say that planning and taking things slowly when you first get onto your property will be crucial in creating and maintaining systems that will stand the test of time.

RAISING ANIMALS

Planning and considering everything that you will need to make your homestead run smoothly is great, but what happens when you want to buy your first animals? Animals can be a tricky investment and I highly recommend that you spend a lot of time researching the proper care for any animals that you want to buy. In the Northeast, three of the best animals to start with on your homestead are chickens, goats, and bees. These animals will thrive in the Northeast climate and can handle the colder winters.

Raising Chickens

The very first step before you buy chicks is to make sure that your city or town allows backyard chickens. Some areas do not permit you to raise chickens. Be sure to check that you have the green light to raise chickens before you purchase any. Don't buy eggs to incubate! Incubating eggs for your first round of chickens is an incredibly delicate process. For inexperienced chicken parents, this process can be needlessly stressful. I recommend buying baby chicks and raising them from when they are young.

Deciding which breed of chickens you want to raise depends on what you want the chickens for. If you want to only have chickens that lay eggs you will want to go with Brahams, Cochins, Orpingtons, or Wyandottes. If you are looking to get eggs and meat from your chickens, you will want to get a dual-purpose breed, such as Barred Rock, Rhode Island Red, Sussex, or White Leghorn chickens. If you are only looking to raise chickens for their meat, I would suggest purchasing Cornish Cross or Red Ranger chicks. Once you have decided on the breed of chicks and purchased them, it is important to keep them extremely warm for the first couple of weeks of their life. Chicks are usually supposed to be with a broody hen that will keep them warm through body heat, and without that they will need a constantly warm environment. Keep the chicks in your home during this period, as a heat lamp in an outdoor coop will not be warm enough. During the first couple of weeks, you will want to line the chick enclosure with pine shavings or a rubber mat so that they aren't slipping around. The chicks will also need chicken feed specifically for chicks, and water.

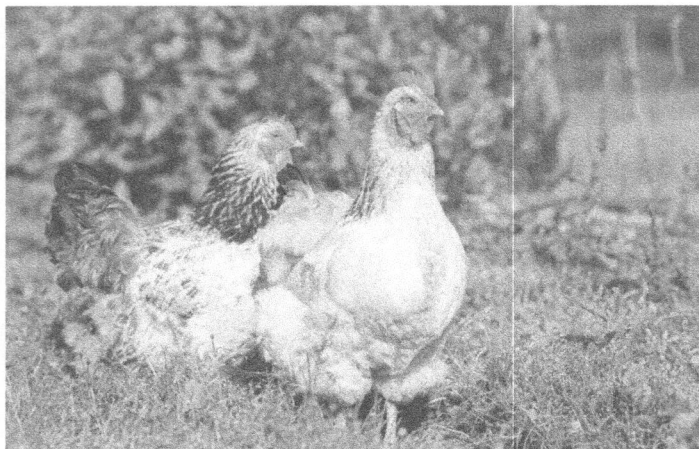

Usually, once the chicks are 8 weeks old, they are ready to be moved to their coop. Be sure to ready to coop with all of the necessary aspects, but leave out any feed or water bowls. Leaving food inside the coop will attract predators and rodents, which you do not want in your coops. Some general precautions to take when you are setting up the chicken coop is to ensure that it remains dry inside the coop to avoid mold, have sturdy latches for all of the doors, and be sure that there is good ventilation throughout the coop. Chickens require some daily chores but other than that, the chores that you will need to complete for your chickens are manageable and can happen on a weekly or monthly basis. Daily, you will want to feed your chickens, make sure they have fresh clean water, and sweep out any droppings that were left overnight. Weekly, you will want to fully clean out the coop and replace the hay. Monthly chores will consist of scrubbing the entire coop, feeds, and water bowls.

The benefits of raising chickens are that you have access to free fertilizer and pest control, organic eggs, and an additional stream of revenue. Collecting the droppings from your chickens is a great way to get organic fertilizer for your gardens. Chickens love to eat bugs and can be used as a great form of pest control for your gardens. However, be careful to note that allowing your chickens unfettered access to your gardens will mean that you will lose some crops, as they are equal-opportunity omnivores. You are also bound to get organic eggs from your chickens if you raise hens. Organic eggs are healthier than store-bought eggs and remove the risk of insecticides and other harmful chemicals. When you collect chicken eggs from your hens, they also don't need to be refrigerated because they were not processed. This can save you a lot of refrigerator space and provides extra time for you to use or sell the eggs. Chicken eggs and meat can be a great source of income for your farm. Depending on the breed of chickens that you raise, you may have access to relatively large organic eggs that other people would love to buy.

Raising Goats

Goats are another easy and manageable animal to raise on your Northeast farm. If you are interested in raising animals for their milk, fiber, or just general companionship, then you may want to invest in some goats. Goats are incredibly personable animals that are easy to care for and will leave a smile on your face every time you are with them. If you are interested in buying goats for their milk, there are five breeds of goats that are perfect for this purpose: Alpines, Nigerian Dwarfs, Nubians, La Manchas, and Saanens.

Alpine goats are great if you are living in an area that gets cold winters, as they do great in cold temperatures. This breed of goat is a medium size and often has really lovely markings. Milking these goats is great for dairy as well as cheese making. Nigerian Dwarfs are small goats that only grow to about 20 inches tall. These goats are great if you don't have excess amounts of land but you want to raise some tiny friends. Nubians are another medium-sized goat breed. They are adorable, kind, and very vocal. If you are starting a homestead with children, Nubians are a great addition to the family. La Manchas are another great option if you are living in the northernmost part of the Northeast as they are relatively cold-hardy animals. The last of the goat breeds to consider for your homestead are Saanens. These goats tend to be large, with calm personalities that are easy for first-time goat owners. However, you will want to have plenty of space on your property for these goats to roam.

Once you have decided what type of goat you'd like to raise, there are some other essentials that your goats will need before they arrive. The goats will need a home, access to clean water, food, and fencing. I recommend that if you are going to raise goats, you either have a property with a barn on it already or build a barn on your farm. In the Northeast specifically, the goats will need a warm place to stay during the winter months. The top priorities for a goat barn are that it is well-ventilated, draft-free, and dry. You will want to keep the barn dry for the same reasons that you will want to keep a chicken coop dry.

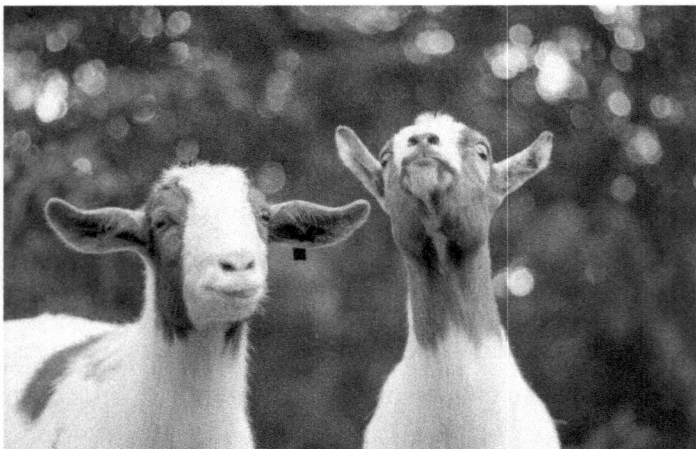

Goats, similar to chickens or any animal that you raise on your farm, need constant access to clean drinking water. This is a relatively inexpensive system to set up but it is important that you consider how you will keep the water from freezing during the winter. There are some heated water bowls that you can use for chickens, but for goats that need a larger water source, a creative option is worth considering. Goats like to browse instead of graze. A goat will hop from food source to food source so that they have variety in their diets. Allowing your goats access to different types of food will leave your goal with a healthier and more well-rounded diet. You can also add hay to their barn for extra food when needed. Woven wire fencing or electric fencing that is tall are the best options if you are raising goats. Goats are smart and inquisitive animals and they will find a way to test your fences if they can. Goats can also jump and climb with ease, so ensure that your fencing is tall if you want to keep your goats inside their enclosure and predators outside of it.

Beekeeping

Raising bees is not only a fulfilling process that will leave you with delicious wild honey, but it is also an act of sustainability. There is a shortage of bees across the United States and without bees the ecological systems in the country will suffer tremendously. If you are considering raising bees, do as much research as you can about keeping bees before you buy a colony. There is a lot of information on bee health and safety that you will need before you can safely start an apiary. It would be heartbreaking if you bought a colony, the colony suffered for some reason that you were unprepared for, and the colony died as a result. Buying colonies can be pretty expensive and if you don't have all the information that you need before you get them, you will waste your money.

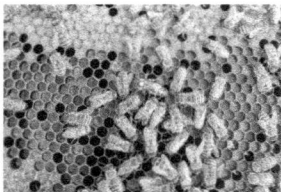

The next step, after you have researched keeping bees, is to get the equipment that you will need. At the most basic level, you will need a beekeeping veil and jacket, gloves, pillars, hive tools, a smoker, and a bee brush. All of these tools are humane to use on the bees and to keep yourself safe while you are handling them. The initial investment in the tools required for beekeeping and one hive will cost a little more than $700 (Melanie, 2020). The best time to order a bee colony is in the winter. Many bee distributors sell out pretty fast, so once you've settled on the bees that you want to keep, be sure to order quickly. Picking a spot to keep your bees is also a crucial step in the process. Bees like to be in spots that are partially shaded and with close access to flowers and other crops that flower for pollination. If the bee hive is kept too far from pollinating flowers, the bees will fly too far and potentially die on the way back to the hive. A weak hive will be targeted by other bees and eventually die as a result.

Once your bees arrive, check the health of your queen bee before you place the bees into the hive. Sadly, without a healthy queen bee, the hive will fail.

Place the hive in your desired location and insert the colony at the beginning of spring. A great tip for the first few weeks of having an active colony is to place some small dishes of sugar water out for the bees. If they are feeding on the sugar water, they are still trying to locate the best flowers. Once they stop feeding from it, they have found flowers and have begun feeding themselves. During the growing season, your beehive won't need too much maintenance. Check the hive once every 2 weeks. Also learn to spot bee eggs. If the queen bee is laying eggs then the hive is thriving! I think that bees are an excellent investment for your first homestead, but similar to many other farming methods and projects, it is critically important that you do as much research on beekeeping as you can. Bees are fragile and need to be cared for by a farmer that knows how to do it.

COMPOSTING

Along the same view of living a self-sustainable life with a focus on healthy practices, composting is another great option for your homestead. Composting is the act of recycling kitchen scraps and other organic materials into a bin. The composting bin should be placed outside of your house and away from direct sunlight. The contents of the bin can be left to mulch over the course of a couple weeks, at which point you can use the mulch as fertilizer for your crops.

Composting has a variety of benefits: not only can you use the composted materials as organic fertilizer for your farm, but you also significantly cut down your own waste production that add to landfills. The fertilizer that you can get from composting is often rich in nutrients that your crops will crave, and you can create luscious gardens out of the composted materials.

In order to begin composting, you will need a shaded area that is away from your home. On a larger property, you want to put your compost in an accessible place that isn't so far from your home that it is a chore to get to. To build a compost bin from scratch, there are many different design options that you can choose from. You can make a compost bin out of a large plastic bin, safe pallet wood, or pieces of wood that have gathered around your farm from other projects. Regardless of the design, it is important that your compost bin has ventilation and a solid latch to avoid any scavengers looking for food. It should also be accessible enough to you that you can add content to the compost bin without hassle. Before you can start regularly adding to your compost bin, you will want to *cold compost*, which is the process of adding leaves, small branches and twigs, newspaper, and kitchen scraps to your compost pile. Be sure to never add any meat or animal products to your compost as that can compromise the integrity and health of your compost pile. Allow all of these materials to break down over the course of a couple of weeks before you begin regularly adding to your compost pile. Cold composting sets the groundwork for a healthy compost bin.

Another aspect to consider when you start composting are the types of materials that you are adding to the bin. There are *brown* materials and *green* materials that will create catalysts for different chemical reactions to occur. Brown materials are leaves, newspaper, or dead grass. The brown materials will supply carbon to your compost bin. Meanwhile, green materials are kitchen scraps, coffee, or fresh grass. The green materials will add nitrogen to your compost bin. Both nitrogen and carbon are essential for a healthy compost bin and generally you will want to add more carbon suppliers or brown material to the compost bin over nitrogen suppliers. The benefits of consciously considering what you are putting in your compost bin will pay off down the line as you are able to create carbon- and nitrogen-rich fertilizer to add to your gardens.

IDEAL PLANT ENVIRONMENTS

Greenhouses

Greenhouses are undoubtedly one of the best environments for your plants to thrive if you are interested in early propagation or growing plants that aren't native to your area. When you are considering building and maintaining a greenhouse on your property, it is important that your greenhouse has adjustable heat, plenty of sunlight, humidity and ventilation control, and as much automation as possible.

There are many different styles of greenhouses that can be built to accommodate exactly what you hope to grow on your farm. There are five aspects to building and maintaining a greenhouse that are essential for your plants' health. The first is the temperature of the greenhouse. As plants are left in a closed space, they will take in CO_2 and release oxygen, which can create a warmer environment if left unattended. There are many ways to control the temperature in your greenhouse through technology, and living in the Northeast, this is definitely an option worth thinking about. If you want to grow crops that would typically struggle to grow in Northeast temperatures, a greenhouse is a perfect solution. Plants like tomatoes, cucumbers, hot peppers, and sweet peas all need a little extra warmth to thrive. As a general rule, you will want the greenhouse on your farm to run north to south so that it gets the most sun that it can during the day. The shelves and crops on the east side of the greenhouse should be lower to the ground and the shelves on the west side should be higher up. This allows the plants to constantly have access to the warmth that they need from the sun.

When considering how much sun your plants want, it may be the case that you have plants in your greenhouse that don't require

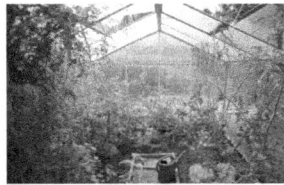

direct sun for long periods of the day. Place these plants either closer to the ground so that there is more chance that they will be shaded or utilize shade covers. I also recommend that if you are building your own greenhouse, you invest in UV-filtering polyethylene plastic. This plastic will filter out any harmful rays and ensure healthier plants all around. As a result of the sunlight and photosynthesis that is occurring in the greenhouse, your greenhouse will become very humid. Humid greenhouses are the ideal environment for many crops that thrive in warm or tropical climates. However, if your greenhouse remains too humid for too long there is a chance that harmful mold or pests can grow. It is important to balance the humidity of the greenhouse with proper ventilation so that you reduce the risk of mold growth. Many of the new construction designs for greenhouses will call for vents to be built directly inside of the greenhouse so that there is constantly proper ventilation. Having solid ventilation is key to fostering the ideal environment for your plants. In the Northeast, there is a chance that the summer months will mean more humidity and it may be worth investing in fans or vents. However, if you are on a budget, adding a couple of hatches into your greenhouse to promote natural ventilation from the wind outside can also be a great option.

The last aspect to building a greenhouse on your property is automation. With the advancement in farming technologies surrounding greenhouses, there are many ways to automate the climate controls, light, and ventilation. To purchase a more automated greenhouse can be quite expensive, but if you are new to farming and have room in your budget for one, I suggest that you go for it. The automations available to you can ensure that you create a thriving environment for your plants to grow with little risk that they won't make it to harvest.

Water and Sunshine

If you are growing in a traditional garden or making use of a greenhouse, it is important to plan out how your plants will be watered. Plants need water in order to grow and for the vast majority of plants, they will take up water through their roots systems. Each plant that you grow will have its own preferences for how often it is watered and the watering cycle will also be affected by the climate. Luckily, in the Northeast, there aren't long periods of drought that you will have to worry about. There will be periods in the summer months when there are heat waves that could jeopardize your plants' health, but with a little extra water and some shade they will make it. When it comes to the daily chore of watering, you can either choose to water by hand using a watering can or hose, which is great for a smaller garden, or you can choose to water your gardens with an irrigation system. For traditional gardens there are underground irrigation systems or sprinkler systems that will work great to automate the watering process. For underground irrigation systems, you will need to invest in some pipes and have a water source that is elevated from where your gardens are. A great practice when you have a water source that is at a higher elevation than your gardens is to allow gravity to do the work for you and feed water through an underground pipe system that will water your crops. For sprinklers, the main hurdle is setting up the technology for them. Supplying water to the sprinklers can come from established water sources on your property, a well, or the county water source that you use to get water in your home. Whichever case works best for you, be sure to plan how you will water your crops and make sure that you are prioritizing that chore when you start on your farm.

Another way to ensure that you create the ideal environments for your plants is to understand the amount of sunlight that they will need. Virtually every plant will need sun in order to grow. During the observation phase, be sure to get a sense of where the sunniest areas are on your property, as well as the ones that get some shade. Each crop will have a preference for how much sunlight that it gets during the day. For traditional gardens in raised beds, find areas that get slightly shaded during the day for the crops that need less than 6 hours of sunlight per day. Similarly, find areas that have access to a lot of sun for the crops that need more than 6 hours of sunlight. In addition to the sunlight that your crops will need, consider your greenhouse as well. If you have a greenhouse on your property, it is important there will be no structures that cause shade on the greenhouse. You can absolutely grow crops in the greenhouse that don't require more than 6 hours of sunlight, but you will need to invest in shade protection if you are looking to do this. When I first built my gardens and greenhouse, I bought a couple of mess shades from Home Depot that were easy to move around my farm. This was a cheap investment that made all of the difference on my property. I was able to move around the shade when I did my daily walks around the farm and as a result, during my first year of growing, I saw incredible results.

Companion Planting

Companion planting is the process of planting different crops near each other because they provide symbiotic relationships to one another. This can be through the way that one crop shades another or how the growing cycles can prevent pests from moving from one crop to the other. In either case, companion planting is a great option when you are first starting your gardens because it provides more access to different crops as well as a healthier garden.

There are endless benefits to companion planting. Some of the benefits include that you save space in your garden, add additional shelter to fragile plants, attract beneficial insects, help maintain nutrient-rich soil, reduce the risks of plant diseases and pest intervention, and cut down on the amount of time you spend weeding.

One of the largest benefits of companion planting is the way that it saves space in your gardens. If you are using the raised-beds technique, you will want to maximize the space that you have in your gardens at all costs. By companion planting you can utilize all of the space in your garden and your crops will thrive as a result. Based on the types of plants that you want to grow using the companion planting method, the plants can provide protection and shade to others. For example, taller plants like tomatoes and beans can provide protection to shorter plants like cabbage and lettuce. Corn stalks can act as a trellis for viney plants. Thus, these companion planting methods can also help you to avoid having to add extra structures into your garden to support smaller crops.

Companion planting can provide great insect control in your gardens. By utilizing specific companion planting methods, you can repel harmful insects and attract beneficial ones. For flying pests that eat at your plants, they will get easily confused by the smell of garlic and onion growing in the garden. Meanwhile, planting Cosmos, black-eyed Susans, and other native flowers can attract ladybugs and other helpful insects that will prey on the harmful insects. Similarly, if you plant diverse native flowers that have varied blooming periods, you will attract bees and butterflies, which are essential pollinators for your garden. For more advanced farmers, you can utilize the trap cropping method, where you plant a perimeter of crops around your garden that attract harmful insects. They will fall for the trap that you have set and not touch the crops that you want to see thrive. Planting collards and Chinese mustard around the perimeter of your yard will attract moths and beetles, while protecting cabbage, spinach, and chard growing in your garden.

Companion planting with nitrogen-efficient crops is a great way to improve your soil quality and allow the plants to share their nutrients. I mentioned earlier that a great way to increase the quality of the soil in your raised beds is to plant cover crops, like ryegrass and clover. This is also a beneficial practice when companion planting because these nitrogen-efficient crops will share their nitrogen with the surrounding crops. There are few crops that can process nitrogen from the air, but by adding a few of these crops into your garden, the soil and other plants will be healthier. Some nitrogen-efficient crops to add to your garden are peas, beans, and any other plant from the legume family. In addition to nutrient sharing, it is also important to rotate your crops between growing seasons. By rotating the nitrogen-rich crops, you can ensure that all of the soil in your garden is nitrogen rich. You can even plant legumes at the end of the season and till them into your soil at the beginning of the spring season for an added nitrogen boost and green compost.

When you are utilizing companion-planting

methods, you will be avoiding monocultures, which are gardens that only grow one type or variety of a plant. These types of gardens are incredibly susceptible to disease and harmful insects. Most gardeners will tell you to avoid monocultures as much as possible. It would be such a headache to buy a ton of seeds for one specific crop that you want to grow, only to see them all be ravaged by insects or fall victim to a disease. By utilizing companion planting, most diseases don't have the ability to fester because of the variety of crops in one area. In addition, weeds will grow in your garden if there is too much space between your crops. For the first growing season, an easy way to avoid excessive weeds is to plant your companion crops close together. You can also try intercropping or sequential cropping. Intercropping calls for planting two crops close together at the same time. This will allow the companion crops to grow at a relatively well-paced rate and avoid competition from weeds. Sequential cropping calls for planting crops sequentially so that there is never a time where there isn't a crop being established. Again, this will cut down on the competition from weeds and decrease the time that you will spend removing weeds from your garden.

There is a resource on *The Old Farmer's Almanac*

website that allows you to plot your gardens using the companion-planting method before you even get started on your property. I highly recommend utilizing this tool to make planting easier down the line. Some examples of companion plants that you may want to incorporate into your garden are:

- Plant marigolds, cosmos, garlic, and onions throughout your gardens to encourage helpful insects to find homes in your garden. Note to keep the garlic and onions away from any beans.
- Basil and tomatoes can be planted together.
- Borage can be planted near tomatoes, strawberries, and squash.
- Basil is a great companion crop for almost every other crop that you can grow in the Northeast.

Some general tips when you start companion planting are to plant short, shade-loving plants beneath taller plants. Be sure to keep tall sun-loving plants on the north end of your garden and short shade-loving plants on the south end. Planting herbs throughout your garden can decrease the number of harmful insects that are attracted to your crops. Plant mint and basil throughout the garden, but. beware that mint grows aggressively and will need to be monitored.

Consider the ideal conditions for every crop. Just because two crops are companions doesn't mean that they need the exact same care. Consider the sun, water, and wind conditions that the individual plants need in order to thrive. Some of these aspects will be negated as a result of companion planting, but you will still need to regularly tend to your garden in order to make the most of a companion-planting method. Also think about the maturation rates for each crop so that you can maximize on space. Planting your crops sequentially based on how long they take to mature can improve the space in your garden and ensure that you have consistent harvests.

MAXIMIZING YOUR YIELD

Before you start working on the farm, there are some steps that you can take to prepare for the season that will maximize your yields. Before the season starts, establish dedicated beds, collect rainwater, plan your beds and choose your crops, and extend the growing season. During the growing season, you will want to nourish the soil, feed your plants what they crave, provide shade to your crops, and take preventative pest-control measures. While these steps may sound like a lot of things to consider, they will start to naturally flow as you get a feel for the growing season.

Establishing dedicated beds for your gardens can be accomplished by setting up your raised beds. I am a personal fan of raised beds because they are versatile and can work on almost any property, so long as you have a sunny spot on which to garden. To take it a step further, you can maximize your yields by automating your raised bed watering systems. There are many raised bed designs that call for irrigation systems and proper drainage that can save you a lot of time that you would otherwise spend watering. Before the growing season starts, you will also want to spend some time collecting rainwater. Rainwater is an incredibly healthy option for your plants, as it will always have the right pH for your crops and is softer than treated water. Rain collection bins are a relatively inexpensive investment that will aid in the growing season. During the off season, set up your rain collection bins so that you have plenty of water stored before the start of the growing season.

Planning your garden beds before the start of the season will also help to maximize your yields. If you have a dedicated plan and you know exactly what you are going to plant where, you will be ultimately more successful during the growing season. I suggest doing as much research as you can about the crops that you want to plant and their preferred conditions, so that you are ready for any obstacle. Use the strategies that I laid out in the companion planting section to do this more efficiently. In Chapters 7, 8, 9, and 10 I will describe the best crops to grow during the three growing seasons in the Northeast, but as a general rule you will want to prioritize growing crops that are native and thrive in your area. Growing crops that are not native to your area will mean that they will have a harder time reaching harvest. For crops that prefer more tropical climates than you are in, use a greenhouse rather than an outdoor garden bed.

Another step to take to maximize your yields before the growing season is to discover when the first and last frost of the year will be. You can plan to extend the growing season each year by putting in plant protections so that you get more harvests during the season. One strategy is to propagate your crops in your greenhouse a couple of weeks before the last frost of the season. Doing this will mean that your crops are ready to be transported outdoors right at the start of the season. You can also invest in cold frames, cloches, and row covers to protect your crops if you are transporting them into your garden when it is still a little chilly outside.

Once the growing season has started you will want to consider your soil and plant nourishment in order to maximize your yield. In the following chapter I will take a deeper dive into maintaining your soil so that you have healthy plants. The general rules for nitrogen-rich soil on your farm will be to use the lasagna compost layering method in your raised beds. Finding every way to ensure that your soil is nitrogen-rich will lead to maximized yields and plenty of harvests. In addition, you can add fertilizer concentrates and natural teas to your crops during the growing season to boost their growing cycles. A great practice, and one that I have utilized in the past, is to grow comfrey near your compost bin. Comfrey is a flowering plant from the borage family that is great to use in fertilizing teas for your crops. The comfrey clippings can also be added to your compost to speed up decomposition, which is great if you are looking to add compost to your gardening beds between seasons.

The last two steps in maximizing your yields are to add shade protection to your gardens and take preventative measures to avoid pests. There are many plants that will thrive in shaded areas and utilizing the shaded areas on your farm can increase the harvests that you reap. Leafy greens and cold-hardy berries will thrive in shaded areas on your farm. I have previously discussed some pest-prevention strategies in your garden. In addition to the strategies, another great tactic to take when trying to prevent pests is to keep the area around your garden clutter-free. Pests will make homes in overturned pots or other small containers and feed on your crops. Maximizing your yields requires an attention to detail for the conditions that your crops will thrive in, and making preemptive efforts will ensure that you are using your space well and providing your garden with adequate support. Following these simple steps will lead to a bountiful garden each and every season.

5

ESSENTIAL SOIL

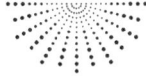

The soil in your garden will be the backbone of the development and health of your plants. It is incredibly important that you understand the soil in your yard and ways to improve the quality of the soil. The four functions of the soil in your garden are to provide a habitat for organisms, provide the foundation for the projects on your farm, recycle raw materials, and be the catalyst for plant growth.

Soil provides water, oxygen, anchorage, temperature modification, and nutrients to your plants. The water added to your soil hydrates the root systems of nearby plants and can cool the plants as the water evaporates from the leaves. This is particularly important if you are growing seasonal crops that require warmer temperatures than are available in the Northeast. Water also carries essential nutrients from the soil into the plants. The oxygen in your soil allows the roots to break down sugars and release energy as part of the photosynthesis cycle. Soil also allows your plants to anchor themselves to the earth. Without soil, the roots system would have nothing to hold on to to support the plant's growth. Soil can also modify the temperature of the roots. The soil can both insulate during cold seasons and provide cooling during the warmer seasons. When you add green compost and other natural fertilizers to your soil, the soil acts as a conductor for those nutrients into the plant's root system. Needless to say, having healthy soil that promotes your plant's growth is crucial to a sustainable garden.

Now that you know why soil is so important, how do you go about finding if your soil is viable and healthy? For the most part, the soil on your property will probably require some intervention when you first get there. Soil that is excessively compacted from foot traffic or vehicles often loses its gardening viability and will need some help. To perform the initial test on your soil, you are going to want to consider the texture, structure, pore space, organic matter, and horticultural capacity. That may seem like a lot but the best way to start a successful garden is with healthy soil

The texture of your soil relates to the amount of sand, silt, and clay in the soil. As a general rule, you want your soil to be 40% sand, 40% silt, and 20% clay. This is hard to determine with the naked eye, but by feeling the soil on your property, you can get a sense of the texture and where to add to your soil to improve it. Next, you want to consider the structure of your soil. It is easy to spot sand in the soil because of its color, but spotting clay and silt is a little tricker. As a general rule, clay and silt stick together to form aggregates. The amount of aggregates in your soil determines the structure of your soil. Higher quality topsoil or loam (the preferred mixture of sand, silt, and clay) is typically granular with few aggregates. If you have good soil structure the soil will have more pore space and promote healthy root penetration. Pore space is the amount of space between the aggregates and other soil components that would allow roots to take hold. As water enters the soil, it creates small pathways that then evaporate as temperatures elevate. These pathways are the perfect homes for roots. Good soil has a combination of large and small porches that provide a balance between the air and water that plants will need during the growing cycle.

The next aspect to consider when you are surveying your soil is the organic matter. Organic matter are the living and organic organisms that you can find in your soil. These could be anything from worms to the leaves that decompose on top of your soil. Having good organic matter can promote water retention and add clay or silt into your soil if it is missing. The horticultural capacity of your soil measures the viability that the soil has to promote healthy plant growth. Good horticultural soil contains 50% soil material, with 5% of that being organic matter and 50% pore space (Berg Stack, 2017). A great way to improve the horticultural capacity of your soil is to irrigate the soil and allow it to drain. If the soil is dry the day after irrigation, it is likely that your soil is dominated by sand. If the soil is wet, there is too much clay in your soil and you need to introduce more organic material to your soil. The best soil ratio for growing vegetables on your farm is a 50:50 ratio between compost and topsoil or loam. The best soil for flowers depends on how you are planting your flowers and the type of flowers you are growing. Flower bulbs thrive in sandy loam soil, and soil mixtures of compost, peat, and topsoil are great for flower gardens from seeds.

The chemical properties of your soil will also come into play when you are observing the viability of the soil on your property. 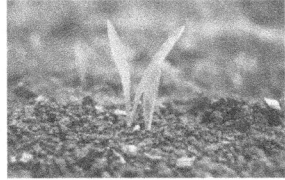 Nitrogen and pH levels are incredibly important to consider when you first start farming. Nitrogen-rich soil allows your plants to thrive as they absorb the nitrogen, which improves their growth cycles. You can add nitrogen to your soil through compost and mulching. The pH levels of your soil are also vitally important because each crop that you plant will have different pH preferences in order to thrive. The pH levels in your soil indicate how acidic or alkaline the soil is. Some plants prefer acidic soil, some prefer alkaline soil, and others prefer base soils. Testing your soil is a great way to get a gauge on how viable your soil will be during the growing season. This process should happen right when you get to your property and before you begin planting. You can test your soil with a pH test that can be purchased at hardware stores or you can mail a sample of your soil to a soil-testing lab. The pH soil testing kits are valuable because they can tell you the pH levels in the soil and there are ways to adjust them. Sending your soil to a soil-testing lab is a great way to get comprehensive information about the pH, texture, nutrients, and other factors in your soil, as well as recommendations for how to treat your soil. The University of Minnesota has a highly esteemed soil testing lab that tests samples from across the country, and their testing prices that start at $17.

Some natural ways that you can improve your soil, maybe while you are waiting for your soil test results, are to till, mulch, and manage the organic matter levels in the soil. You can also naturally alter the pH levels of your soil. Tilling your soil will loosen the soil and add aeration and pores. This is great because it allows more root systems to become established and provides space for you to add other soil components. Mulching your soil is the process of adding organic composted materials, which introduces more nitrogen and organic matter. Mulch also helps to retain warmer temperatures and moisture. If you add mulch to your soil you can also decrease weed growth and harmful insect presence. Introducing and managing the organic matter levels can additionally improve the soil quality. Adding leaves so that they can decompose will introduce new organic matter into the soil. Alternatively, you could start a worm farm so that there are plenty of earth-worms paving new root pathways in your soil. The more you manage the organic matter, the more fertile and long-lasting your soil viability will be.

Improving your soil pH through natural means will look very similar to the previously listed ideas for how to improve your soil. Adding organic matter, maximizing the drainage and air exposure that your soil gets, keeping the soil covered, avoiding chemical interventions, and rotating crops will all lead to more sustainable pH levels. Adding organic matter will improve the pH because of the chemical interactions that organic matter introduces. Worms can be a great way to change the pH levels of your soil as they add new matter that will alter the pH to be more basic. Worms and other organic matter can also create more air and water exposure and improve the drainage that your soil has. This is great if you are looking to get more alkaline pH levels. Keeping your soil covered with leaves and mulch can also improve the pH because the natural erosion that soil will encounter when left exposed to the elements will alter the pH. Covering the soil will give you more control over the soil pH and intro-duce nitrogen-richness.

I don't know about you, but when I started the

self-sustaining homestead journey, I was determined to find natural solutions to farming projects. Adding chemical pesticides and other soil treatments seemed to go against this goal. Not only do I have no idea what the chemical interactions will do to my soil, but I was also nervous that all of the hard work that I was doing to improve the soil pH would be undone. Stay away from chemical pesticides and other treatments because they can in fact alter the soil pH and damage your plants. There are different remedies to intercept harmful insects that don't require chemicals. You also don't want to indiscriminately remove all insects from your garden. There are many helpful insects that can promote healthy plant growth in your garden and fertilize different areas.

The last way to improve your soil pH is by rotating your crops between growing seasons. If you have perennial crops planted in one area, it is fine to let them stay in that area, but for the crops that you transported inside, find a new home for them the following spring. Rotating your crops from garden bed to garden bed will introduce new soil conditions and lead to an overall healthier soil across your garden.

The role of fertilizer and adding your compost to

your soil is another way that you can improve the soil. Composting can increase your self-reliance and establish a system on your farm that can be beneficial to your crops. However, I would be remiss if I didn't outline the difference between *mineral* and *organic* fertilizers. So far, I have been promoting the idea of organic fertilizers. Organic fertilizers consist of composted materials that you collect on your farm. The benefits of composting are that the compost can add much needed nutrients to your soil and promote self-sustainable practices. However, composting takes a while to decompose and you need to be very conscious of what you are putting in the compost. The goal of composting to add to your soil is that you are providing the soil with the correct balance of nutrients that it needs. There are 17 different nutrients that plants need to thrive in a garden; if you are not considering what you are putting in your compost, it is possible that you will miss some of those key nutrients.

On the other hand, you can consider mineral fertilizers. Typically, farmers utilize mineral fertilizers when they have extensive farms that they simply can't supply with compost. Mineral fertilizers add all of the necessary nutrients that plants need and can be purchased. The benefits of mineral fertilizers is their convenience and balance. You won't have to consider the nutrients in mineral fertilizers because they are all there. Whichever you choose is a matter of preference. For smaller gardens, conscious composting is definitely the way to go and it will save you money. For larger homesteading operations, it may be worth taking a look at getting some mineral fertilizers.

Regardless of the fertilizing method that you choose, it is also important to note that whatever you put in your fertilizer will come back to you through consumption. If you go the natural fertilizer route, keep in mind what types of things you are adding to your compost pile. Those nutrients will be present in the crops that you harvest. If you go the mineral fertilizer route, be sure to research the type of mineral fertilizer and the minerals that you are putting into your soil. These minerals and the nutrients that they provide will also show up in your food.

6

INCORPORATING PERMACULTURE

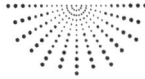

*P*ermaculture stands for permanent culture or permanent agriculture. The permaculture design method is one that prioritizes how your farm will work as one cohesive unit with permanent structures that support your agriculture. One of the founders of the permaculture design strategy said that permaculture is the integrated design system that's modeled on nature (April, 2016). A perfect permaculture design would mean that the systems you've set up around your property perfectly manage the other systems with limited interference from things that exist outside of nature. At its core, permaculture is a system that promotes self-reliance and sustainability.

Incorporating permaculture into your gardens

calls for four types of gardening: companion planting, raised beds or vertical gardening, edible gardening, and keyhole gardening. Companion planting
and raised beds, as already discussed, are my
personal preference and systems that have worked
exceptionally well for myself and others. In addition
to those two types of gardening, there is also an
option to vertical garden. Vertical gardening is typically used in smaller spaces to conserve the amount
of square feet needed to build and maintain a
garden. Permaculture gardening also calls for edible
gardening. Edible gardens are often called 'kitchen
gardens' or 'survival gardens.' This is the practice of
gardening for self-sustainability. You eat and serve
what you harvest from your gardens in an effort to
be reliable and sustainable. Keyhole gardening,
much like raised beds or vertical gardening, is a
different style of gardening that calls for horseshoe-
shaped gardens. This style of gardening promotes
companion planting and helps to cultivate both
perennial and annual plants. All of these gardening
techniques can be combined on your property or
you can modify the techniques so that they adjust to
the space that you have available on your farm.

ETHICS AND PRINCIPLES OF PERMACULTURE DESIGN

When you are implementing permaculture design into your farm, there are three ethics that permaculture design is based on. Upholding these three ethics will inevitably lead you toward a more productive farm and a cultivated community to enjoy it. The first ethic is care for the Earth. Caring for the Earth calls for the careful consideration of the land that you are interacting with, as well as care for all living and nonliving things that inhabit the Earth. It can also be called conscious consumerism. Permaculture design calls for taking care of the Earth so that it will thrive under natural circumstances and consuming foods and products that are also made with the care of the Earth in mind. The second ethic is caring for people. Caring for people calls for the maintenance of all of the basic needs that people have to be met. Food, shelter, water, education, employment, and socialization are all aspects of caring for people that should simply be given without the promotion of status or wealth. While this may seem like a far-fetched idea that is rooted in idealism, the importance of caring for people when you are living on a farm can start small. Ensuring that all of the basic needs for you and your family are met is adhering to the caring for people ethic of permaculture design. Hopefully, once you have established the ethic for yourself and your family, you can broaden your scope to other people in your community. The third and final ethic of permaculture design is fair shares. This ethic combines the ideologies of the first two. It is pointless to engage in caring for the Earth and caring for people if there is not an expectation that everyone is entitled to the same level of care. Fair shares call for everyone having access to their basic needs and giving back to the Earth in a sustainable way.

Beyond the three ethics that underpin the ideas of permaculture design, the founders of the design system also create the 12 principles of permaculture design. The first principle of permaculture design is to observe and interact with the Earth and others. The more we observe the world around us, the more we will be able to consciously interact with it. This is also a great way to learn from your environment about its needs. You may be sitting out in your garden and observing the slope in your lawn. You can see how the organic shapes of the land inform the best way to grow crops in those areas.

The second principle is to catch and store energy.

Ultimately, permaculture design is geared toward off-the-grid living. This doesn't necessarily mean living in isolation, but rather living as self-reliantly as possible. Collecting energy from the wind or sun is a great way to begin this process. You can also collect other renewable resources to generate energy on your property, like rainwater or the energy from a rushing river.

The third principle is to obtain a yield. Planting and cultivating crops in an effort to be self-sustainable is one of the central tenets to permaculture design. However, this principle has a hidden agenda. The more time that you spend outside, the happier and at peace you will feel with your environment.

The fourth principle is to apply self-regulation and feedback on your homestead. In a world that is facing drastic consequences as a result of climate change, it is important to center sustainable changes into your permaculture design. The goal of the fourth principle is to reduce your negative impacts on the Earth and note where you can do better.

The fifth principle is to use and value renewable resources. Again, this principle is calling for a more sustainable lifestyle. Switch away from non-renewable resources and prioritize renewable options. We already have all of the skills to use renewable resources in our day-to-day lives but because of convenience, we have overlooked more sustainable options. It is time to go back to the renewable options if we want to prolong the life of the planet.

The sixth principle is to produce no waste. I mentioned earlier that permaculture design foundationally calls for using everything on your farm for multiple purposes. Composting and recycling materials that you collect on your farm will make it so that you can adhere to the sixth principle with ease.

The seventh principle of permaculture design is to design from patterns to details. I am a very detail-oriented person and when I first discovered homesteading, I was determined to create multiple options and ways of designing a farm. I spent weeks thinking about all of the materials I would need to buy, ways that I could use the land around me to support different projects, and the impacts that those projects would have on the Earth. I soon learned that actually being on the farm made all the difference. Some days are harder than others and that can lead to convenience being more tempting than sustainability. However, I learned that prioritizing designing from the broad ideas down to little details made the process much easier. It is easier to plan for all of the little things when you take your time and know exactly what you are working on and how it will impact the land.

The eighth principle is to integrate and avoid segregation. The best example of segregation in your garden is planting a monoculture. To adhere to permaculture design, you want to be enriching the earth and giving back. A monoculture limits your ability to do this and comes with a high failure rate. Instead of planting a monoculture, plant a polyculture: a garden that has many different crops growing that support one another and the ecosystem around them. This can be applied to many other areas of homesteading as well. Get invested with the community around you and don't rely on isolation.

The ninth principle is to practice small and slow solutions. By going slow and working on pieces of different projects on your farm, you will be able to remedy issues in a way that doesn't disrupt the ecosystem that you are cultivating. Going fast and large with your projects can mean causing undue chaos on areas of your farm and potentially risk the integrity of the other systems you have created. This principle also applies to starting new projects. Diving head first into new projects can leave space for mistakes that may cause you or your farm harm. Take it slow and ask a lot of questions!

The tenth principle is to use and value diversity. I have said this before, but growing a monoculture garden is bound to lead to issues. With a polyculture garden, the diversity of produce as well as the overall impact on your ecosystem is far more beneficial. The nature on your farm is bound to thrive if you value the diversity of your area and make all of the aspects of your farm work in tandem.

The second to last principle is to use edges and value the marginal. Thinking creatively and problem solving on your farm to fit your specific needs will demonstrate much higher yields for your farm than taking routes that are well established. Of course there are well-established means for developing a farm, but you will need to fit them to your situation. Discover the marginal ways that you can problem solve or integrate new systems into your farm that may be less well established, or take a creative spin on an established farming technique.

The last principle for permaculture design is to creatively use and respond to change. This principle ties together a lot of the ideas that permaculture design espouses. Taking a holistic approach to your farm will allow you to observe and intervene in different areas at the right time instead of forcefully implementing new systems. You want to be creatively working with the organic ecosystem around you.

Permaculture Zones

Within permaculture design, when you are ready to start planning the layout of your farm, there are five zones to consider. The permaculture zones are general guidelines for the layout of your farm so that each zone is accessible and functional within your ecosystem. Zone 0 is your house. This zone is all of the systems that you set up inside of your house to benefit your experience on the farm. Whatever you want to have in your home to make you comfortable and lead to a more sustainable life will be part of zone 0. The next is zone 1. Everything in zone 1 is immediately outside of your house. The elements in zone 1 are things that need daily attention. Your zone 1 could include a kitchen garden, an area to enjoy lunch outside, or a small kitchen coop. The goal of zone 1 is for it to be immediately accessible to you once you step out of our house. The systems in zone 1 should be those that require regular attention and maintenance. You wouldn't want to put your chicken coop 10 minutes away from your front door if you have to go there every day.

Zone 2 is the farming zone. This zone will also require daily attention but there should be an emphasis on a well-integrated system. Your larger gardens and crops should be growing in zone 2, with an irrigation system and access to fertilizer and compost. Zone 2 can also be an area where animals are housed. Chickens, rabbits, ducks, and other animals are great to place in zone 2, as you will regularly visit them and set up systems for them that can be maintained a couple times a week.

Zone 3 is reserved for larger animals and seasonal crops. Larger animals will do great in zone 3 because there is more space for them to selectively graze and fertilize seasonal crops with their droppings. Having a large annual crop garden in zone 3 is also a great option because they don't need consistent care. You will need to have an integrated system for irrigation and maintenance as you may not be visiting it regularly.

Zone 4 is the home orchard, forest, and foraging zone. If you are looking to start an orchard, zone 4 is a great place to put it. Orchards do not require daily maintenance and can provide some snacks for your grazing animals. Zone 4 is also great as a forest for collecting wood or setting up a coppicing operation.

The last zone is zone 5, your wildlife zone. This

zone should remain relatively untouched. This is a great place to observe nature and see how the ecosystem around your farm interacts.

The zones are a guideline to create a well-integrated farm that works on a feedback loop. You will want everything on your farm to serve multiple purposes, and by following the permaculture zones, you can accomplish this much more easily. It is important to note that many properties are not large enough to reach zones 4 and 5. That is perfectly acceptable. You don't have to have every zone on your farm for it to be successful. The goal is to use what you have and work with the nature around you.

Benefits and Drawbacks

One of the benefits to permaculture gardening is that nothing is wasted. Everything has multiple purposes and can be used to cultivate your garden. If I get an early frost on my Northeast farm and some of my plants are shocked and can no longer be harvested, I place the plants into my compost bin. Once the plants have decomposed, I use that compost as additional nutrients in the soil for the following growing season. In addition to the benefits of not wasting anything on your farm, permaculture farming also improves that quality of your gardens. I have discussed some of the methods for collecting water and promoting healthy insect intervention in your gardens. These principles all stem from permaculture design. You want to create a small ecosystem in your garden that is self-sustaining. By recycling rain water and planting flowers that will attract helpful insects, your garden will thrive under conditions that it would if it were growing in the wild.

Inversely, one of the drawbacks to permaculture design is working with what you have. If you buy a property that isn't conducive to a specific type of energy storage or farming technique, you need to roll with the punches. Finding creative solutions can be an exhaustive process where you spend days or weeks racking your brain for the right way to work with the nature around you. Creative solutions can also mean that you are developing new systems on your farm a lot slower than people who opt out of permaculture design. However, the ecological benefits from following permaculture design methods will mean that your systems will ultimately be healthier for yourself and the planet, with long-lasting results. People who opt out of permaculture often find themselves fighting against nature rather than working with it.

PERENNIAL AND ANNUAL PLANTS

Now that you understand the basics of permaculture design, it is time to consider the best plants to grow in your garden. There are two categories of plants that you can grow: perennial and annual. Perennial plants are those that are seeded in the spring and will regrow each year without much intervention. Annual plants are plants that are seeded in the spring but die at the end of the growing season. Annual plants need to be replanted each year. As a bonus, there are also biennial plants, which are seeded at the beginning of spring and will seed again the following spring, but they won't be ready to harvest until the end of the second growing season. Most biennials will drop seeds at the end of their growing cycle and in another two growing seasons, they will be ready for harvest again.

In general, it is common for most gardeners to use a combination of both perennial and annual plants in their gardens. In the Northeast, depending on how cold it gets in the winter, you can grow almost any annual plant in your garden or greenhouse with the added benefit that you don't have to worry about it surviving the winter. Perennial plants in the Northeast must be cold-hardy so that they can survive the winter months and regrow the following spring. The combination of perennial and annual plants that you chose to grow is a matter of preference. In the following chapters, I will discuss the best perennial and annual crops to grow in each season on a Northeast homestead.

7

SPRING

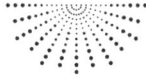

n the Northeast, there are specific steps that you will need to take on your farm to prepare and thrive during each season. From February to May, as the frost clears, it is time to take those initial steps to set up your farm for a productive year. The first step is to inspect your farm. If this is your first year on the farm, take note of any cold or ice damage that has been left on the farm from the winter. Be sure that all of your raised beds are clean and remove any frost that may be covering them. Next, take a look at the exterior of the existing structures on your farm. Do any walls or windows have cold damage, chips, or leaks? Be sure that all of your existing structures are repaired before you dive into preparing for the growing season. Once your farmhouse, barns, and other structures are patched up, move on to spring cleaning. Rake out any dead foliage and be sure that the area for your raised beds is cleared.

Having a clean farm to start the season will mean less chaos later in the season. On my first farm, I didn't patch up some of the walls on my house that bordered my kitchen garden. Before I knew it, I had some vines growing up and into my house. While I thought it was pretty, it became more of a nuisance than anything else. I patched up the holes in the summer and learned from the experience. You can avoid my mistake by taking stock of your property before the start of the growing season. The next couple of steps are to set you up best to start growing. Test your soil, adjust as needed, and prune any trees or shrubs that have overgrown. The importance of testing and adjusting your soil cannot be understated. As discussed in Chapter 5, starting the growing season with nitrogen-rich soil will maximize your yield and lead to less plant death throughout the year. You can also add the clippings from your trees and shrubs to your compost for nitrogen-rich compost that you can add to your raised beds in a later season.

Before you begin planting your seedlings into your raised beds, be sure to divide your perennial and annual seeds so that you can maximize your yield and not accidentally unearth a perennial plant. Now you can lay out your raised beds and place any stakes or trellises necessary for the specific plants that you are growing. Be sure to grab some extra protective resources for your outdoor garden in case of any cold nights, to avoid plant death at the start of the season if there's a late frost. The listed vegetables that you can grow in the spring are relatively cool-hardy crops that will wither on hot days or nights. To avoid having them suffer through hotter temperatures, plant these vegetables in the early spring so that you can harvest them before the summer. These same crops can also be planted in late summer and fall due to the cooler temperatures.

SPRING VEGETABLES

The ideal vegetables to grow on your farm during the first half of spring are peas, onions, radishes, spinach, lettuce, and turnips. Each of these crops has specific conditions that need to be met so that they can thrive. These vegetables can generally be planted in some Northeast farm regions during the week of

Valentine's Day in February. However, for more northern regions in the Northeast, the first couple of weeks in February is when you want to start your seeds indoors. Of these vegetables, peas, radishes, spinach, lettuce, and turnips are annual and onions are perennial. When you are ready to get started in the spring, follow these steps to get the best yield from your vegetable garden.

All of the following plants can be directly planted outside in February in any Northeast region not still under snow. Plant peas 1 inch into the soil at least 2 inches from other crops. Peas will take at least 60 days to reach their first harvest. Water your peas once to twice a week. Peas are companion plants with green beans, cucumbers, lettuce, squash, and corn. Onions should be planted ½ inch into the soil at least 4 inches from surrounding crops. They will take anywhere from 60 to 90 days for their first harvest, depending on the variety. Water your onions once a week. Onions are companion plants with radishes, carrots, and tomatoes. Plant radish seeds ¼ inch into the soil at least 3 inches from surrounding crops. Radishes will reach their first harvest in 35 days. They need to be watered once to twice a week. Companion plants to keep near radishes are green beans, cucumbers, lettuce, and squash.

Spinach seeds should be planted a ½ inch into the soil. Be sure that the spinach seeds are at least 4 inches from other crops. They will take 35 days to reach their first harvest and will need to be watered once to twice a week. Plant your spinach near radishes, peppers, and tomatoes. Plant lettuce ¼ inch into the soil at least a ½ foot from other crops. Lettuce will take 45 days to reach its first harvest. Water your lettuce once to twice a week. Companion plants to keep near lettuce are tomatoes, cucumbers, onions, garlic, and radishes. The last crop to plant in this round is turnips. Plant turnips ¼ inch into the soil with at least 6 inches away from other crops. Turnips will be ready to harvest 35 days after they are planted and only need to be watered once a week. Turnips are companion plants to broccoli, Brussels sprout, and cabbage.

Along with the previously listed plants, the following can also be planted in February but they should be started indoors. Of these plants, broccoli, cauliflower, and cabbage are annual and Brussels sprout are biennial plants. Plant broccoli and Brussels sprout ¼ inch into the soil at least a foot or two from other crops. They take around 50 days to reach their first harvest. Water your broccoli and Brussels sprout once to twice a week. Plant your broccoli and Brussels sprout near green beans and lettuce. Cabbage and cauliflower should also be planted ¼ inch into the soil and you can expect your first harvest at least 60 days after they are planted. Both crops need to be watered at least once a week. You can plant your broccoli, Brussels sprout, cauliflower, and cabbage seeds indoors from March 27th through April 10th, or you can plant the seedlings outdoors in the following 2 weeks. As a general rule, the leafy green crops can be in more shaded areas of your garden, while the other vegetables want more access to the sun.

The second round of spring vegetables consist of beets, carrots, Swiss chard, potatoes, and parsnips. These plants can generally be planted in the last 2 weeks of May or early April. All of the second-round crops only need to be watered once a week. Beet seeds should be planted ½ inch into the soil with at least 4 inches between them and surrounding crops. Beets will have their first harvest 45 days after planting. Carrots and parsnips should be planted ¼ inch into the soil with 3 inches between seeds. Carrots will harvest 60 to 70 days after planting and parsnips will take at least 105 days to reach their first harvest. Plant your Swiss chard seeds ½ inch into the soil with at least 4 inches between the seeds and surrounding crops. Swiss chard will take at least 50 days to reach its first harvest. You can get a headstart with your Swiss chard seeds by propagating the seeds indoors between April 10th and 24th. The seedlings should be ready to be moved outdoors during the first week of May. Potatoes need to be planted 6 inches into the soil with at least a foot of space between the seeds and surrounding crops. Potatoes will take at least 70 days to reach their first harvest.

SPRING FRUITS AND HERBS

Due to the frosts in the Northeast, fruits and herbs are a little difficult to grow early in the season. Mint, nettles, thyme, oregano, and strawberries are all great options to plant later in the spring season. These plants will suffer if exposed to frost. Mint plants only need partial-sun exposure, so they are great for the more shaded areas of your garden. Mint should be planted toward the end of the spring season or the beginning of summer. Be sure to leave at least a foot of space between mint and other crops, as it is an aggressive grower. Water your mint plants at least once a week for the best results. Nettles, like many of the spring vegetables, should be started indoors about 6 weeks before the last frost. Nettle seeds should be planted ¼ inch into the soil and need to be watered at least once a week. Your first harvest will come 80 days after you transplant the nettles outdoors. Wear gloves when you are harvesting nettles as they have tiny hairs that can get embedded under your skin and cause allergic reactions.

Plant thyme at least 4 weeks into the spring season, as they cannot withstand any frosty nights. Thyme plants need to be planted at least a foot from other crops and they want to be in full-sun areas of your garden. Water your thyme plants at least once a week. Oregano can be planted along-side thyme with similar harvest times. Oregano is an aggressive grower, so be sure to prune the leaves after the first harvest to avoid it taking over areas of your garden. Strawberries are a great spring fruit to put into your raised beds. Strawberries need to have at least 18 inches between surrounding crops when planted. Water your strawberries every week for the best results. The best time to harvest your strawberries is early in the morning and place them directly in your refrigerator to preserve their freshness.

SPRING FLOWERS

There are many different flowers that you can grow in the Northeast, as many of them require planting bulbs at the end of fall that will blossom in the spring. Flowers are a great option for your gardens because they attract helpful insects and can bring a vibrancy that will leave you feeling serene each time you tend to your garden. Daffodils, grape hyacinth, and pansies are three great options when you are considering flowers for your Northeast homestead garden.

Daffodils are full-sun flowers that need access to plenty of sun and water during the growing season. If you are growing daffodil bulbs, you can plant the bulbs 2 to 4 weeks before the ground freezes in the fall. Daffodils won't spread too far in your garden and you can harvest daughter bulbs from your initial bulbs when you harvest the daffodils. As a general rule, if you are planting bulbs, they want to be planted two times deeper in the soil than they are tall. Daffodils need to be watered regularly or they may wither and die. You can only plant grape hyacinths as bulbs at the end of fall. These beautiful flowers are sure to bring vibrant life to your garden. Grape hyacinths are aggressive growers and should be kept at a decent distance from other crops so that they don't take over an area. Don't be scared if you see grape hyacinth leaves breach the soil during the fall; they are cold-hardy bulbs that will blossom in the spring. Once the hyacinths blossom, they don't need excessive watering and often do just fine from rainwater. Pansies are full-sun flowers that will grow all year if treated well. However, unlike daffodils and grape hyacinths, pansies are annual flowers that will need to be replanted each spring. I recommend for your first growing season to buy established pansies instead of trying to start from seeds, as they are very delicate and can easily die during propagation. When you plant your pansies, be sure to leave about 12 inches of space between the flowers and other crops. Pansies need to be regularly watered and maintained as they are susceptible to many harmful insects and mold. With a little extra care, your garden will be full of a rainbow of pansies.

Some other flowers to consider adding to your garden are English daisies, nemesia, twinspur, Icelandic poppies, monkey flower, fritillaries, snowdrops, and violets. All of these flowers fare well in the Northeast. English daisies are a great addition to your spring gardens because they bring added vibrancy to your raised beds and they will blossom at the start of spring. It is important to note that these daisies are aggressive growers and should be contained in a raised bed so that they are more manageable. They are also partial-sun biennial flowers that will not blossom the first year that you plant them but will come into full bloom the second year that they are in your raised beds. Place your English daisies in the shadier spots on your farm that need a little extra color. Nemesia is an annual flower that you can add to your garden that is very low maintenance. For beginners, buy your nemesia plants or bulbs from a nursery if you'd like to add them to your garden, as they usually don't do well if transported into a garden as seedlings. Plant your nemesia bulbs before the first frost in the fall and wait for them to bloom in late spring. They do well in cooler temperatures, so if your farm gets too hot in the summer, it is best to keep these flowers in a slightly shaded spot.

If you are looking to add flowers to your garden that will attract helpful insects that will pollinate your garden, consider planting twinspur. Twinspur are tall flowering plants that can act as a companion plant to those that are low to the ground and require more coverage. They will thrive in full-sun spots in your garden and need to be watered at least once a week. Twinspur can be planted directly into the soil of your raised beds at the end of spring, once temperatures have risen and there is no more risk of frost. Another flower to add to your gardens that will attract helpful insects are Icelandic poppies. These poppies thrive best in later spring and early summer. Icelandic poppies need to be planted in late fall in order to blossom in the spring. Be sure to keep these poppies in full-sun areas and water occasionally; rainwater will most likely do the trick. Try your best not to transplant these flowers to other areas in your garden once they begin to germinate, as they don't fare well during transport.

If you enjoy planting bulbs in the late fall to see a blossoming garden in the spring, add fritillaria flowers to your garden. Depending on the variety of fritillaria flowers that you plant, they can either thrive in shaded raised beds or full-sun raised beds with good soil drainage. The bulbs should be planted in fall, around September or October, for the best results. Fritillaria may attract unwanted beetles, slugs, and snails to your garden and it is best to remove the insects by hand if you encounter them to discourage their presence in your garden beds.

Many Northeast properties will have natural water structures running through the farm or areas that get damp after rainfall. If you have an area like that on your property, consider planting monkey flowers there. Monkey flowers are great Northeast flowers as they are cold-hardy and will attract native butterflies to your garden. These flowers want to be started indoors during the last few weeks of winter and the first weeks of spring. They can be planted at the start of spring and still thrive if there is frost. Once temperatures rise, they will begin to blossom if they are planted in partial-sun raised beds on your farm. A similar flower that will thrive in colder temperatures are snowdrops. Snowdrops are sold as bulbs and should be planted in the fall. These flowers will blossom very quickly and add life to your garden during the winter months. They are also pest-resistant. If you are creating a perimeter garden to ward off unwanted insects and critters, plant snowdrops to keep them away. Be sure to keep your snowdrops in well-draining soil in shaded areas. Snowdrops will become dormant in the spring but they will blossom again in the fall.

Finally, if you are looking for a low maintenance

flower that can add color to your garden, violets are the way to go. Wild violets have a tendency to grow aggressively and spread quickly across your farm so be sure to place them in a raised bed to control their growth. Violets are very self-sustainable and will seed the ground without any intervention. They can be planted in virtually any condition and only need rainwater to thrive.

8
SUMMER

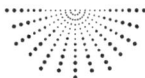

The spring season is always going to be one of the busiest seasons of the year because you will be preparing for a whole year of growing. In the summer months, from June to August in the Northeast, you have time to refine your gardens and add new crops into place as your spring plants come to harvest. After your first harvests from your spring crops, it is time to do some light maintenance of your farm. Go into your raised beds and remove any weeds or dead leaves. Add a new layer of mulch to the garden beds and put in new supports to any plants that may need the helping hand. Treat any harmful pest problems or diseases that may have arisen during the spring. Once you have taken care of the summer cleaning, you can move on to sequentially planning new summer crops.

If you haven't done so already, at the start of the summer is a great time to place aeration tubes in your raised beds. Aeration tubes will bring water directly into the root system. These are a great stop measure to ward against any droughts or heat waves during the summer months.

SUMMER VEGETABLES

At this point in the year you will start to see great yields from the spring growing season and you will feel driven to continue planting. Many of the spring vegetables can be replanted or you can continue to plant them into the summer. The best summer vegetables to add to your Northeast garden are cucumbers, peppers, pumpkins, summer and winter squash, tomatoes, and corn. These vegetables can be started indoors or after the last frost on your property. All of the summer vegetables are annual and will require replanting each season. Cucumbers need to be planted ½ inch into the soil and about 6 inches from other crops. Your first cucumber harvest will come at least 45 days after they are first planted. Cucumbers need to be watered every week.

Peppers do best when they are planted ¼ inch into the soil and at least a foot from other crops. Peppers will come to harvest after 65 days from when they are first planted. Peppers don't require weekly watering and will do fine with rainwater and bi-weekly watering.

Pumpkin seeds can be planted in shallow ditches in your raised beds, about ¾ of an inch into the soil. Pumpkins need a lot of space and should have 3 to 4 feet between their seeds. After you plant your pumpkins, you can expect harvests after 85 days of growing. Pumpkins, like peppers, don't require constant watering. Summer and winter squash should be planted in the same way that pumpkins are. Winter squash require 4 feet between surrounding crops. Summer squash will be ready to harvest 45 days after planting and winter squash will be ready after 85 days. Both squashes require semi-regularly watering: once a week to every other week. Tomatoes also want to be planted ¼ inch into the soil with at least 2 feet between the tomato seeds and other crops. Tomatoes will be ready to harvest after 65 days if they are watered once a week. Corn is very susceptible to frost and will not grow if temperatures drop too low. In the summer, try sowing the corn every 2 weeks for 6 weeks to get the best yields.

Be sure to keep the corn crops about 10 inches from one another. Plant your corn 1 inch deep in moist summer soil. Be careful with the corn roots as they are very fragile during the growing phase. Also take care of any weeds in the area as they can also disrupt the corn roots.

SUMMER FRUITS AND HERBS

The summer is a great time to get all of the delicious fruits and herbs into your raised beds and orchard. The best fruit to plant in the summer are apples, blueberries, cherries, melons, peaches, raspberries, cantaloupe, nectarines, pears, plums, and watermelon. You can also replant any herbs from the spring that were struggling or that you want more of in your kitchen, in addition to basil.

In general, fruit trees need a lot of sun and a lot of space. Plant your fruit tree saplings in the earliest weeks of the summer so they have plenty of time to root during the growing season. Be sure to leave a well around the base of the fruit tree so that the roots get well watered when you irrigate them. Stake your trees when they are still small to support their growth. Be sure to mulch your fruit trees often when they are growing. Trees soak up a lot of nutrients from the soil, as well as water, and will need a lot of attention during the early phases of growth. Great fruit trees to grow on a Northeast farm are apples, cherries, nectarines, peaches, pears, and plums. Each of these trees follows the previously mentioned guidelines, with some exceptions. Be sure to research the right fruit trees for your area, as prioritizing native fruit trees will ensure their success.

Berry bushes also want to be planted in the early part of the summer for the highest yield. Blueberries and raspberries are a great option for virtually every Northeast homestead. Be sure to test your soil pH before planting a berry bush, as they are very susceptible to the pH levels in the soil. If the pH isn't right, you might want to plant your berry bushes in raised beds so that you can have more control over the soil. Raspberry bushes will particularly thrive if they are planted near garlic and onions.

Melons, cantaloupe, and watermelons are also summer fruits that can be grown during the first few weeks of summer. Melons can actually be planted toward the end of spring but will fare just fine when planted in the summer. Be sure to give your melons plenty of space to spread out during their growing cycle. Melons, cantaloupes, and watermelons are full-sun plants that love moist, well-draining soil.

Cantaloupe is not very cold-sensitive but water-melons and honeydew can wither if they are exposed to frosts. Be sure to plant your melons, cantaloupes, and watermelons at least 2 feet apart in raised beds that are at least 6 feet away from other beds. Wherever you choose to plant your melons, it is important to regularly add nutrients to their soil as the leaves of the melon plants will add extra sugars into the soil. To balance out this interaction, regularly add compost, mulch, and other organic fertilizers to the raised beds that are housing the melons. To ensure that your melons are getting the proper water that they need, add a soaker hose or drip system to your melons. They need constant moisture in order to thrive; however, stop watering the crops once they begin to ripen as the excess water will make the melons taste bitter. All three melon types mature at different rates but they will assuredly yield great harvests when treated well. As a general rule, your melons will be ready to harvest when the rind becomes soft and the melons produce a sweet smell in your garden. If you knock on the melon rind and hear a hollow sound, they are ready to be harvested.

SUMMER FLOWERS

The summer is also a great time to add more color to your garden. Zinnias, four o'clocks, marigolds, nasturtiums, cosmos, and sunflowers will be perfect additions to your raised beds. All of the summer flowers are annual and will not rebloom in the spring. Zinnias will attract butterflies to your garden, which are helpful insects to have around, especially if you are growing in raised beds. Butterflies will help pollinate the surrounding flowers and even the vegetables that have a flowering stage. There are three types of zinnias to choose from for your garden, all of which will attract butterflies: single-flowered, double-flowered, and semi double-flowered zinnias. The difference between the three types is purely aesthetic and indicates the amount of petal rows that will be visible at the center of the zinnia. Plant your zinnia seeds directly into your garden beds in a permanent location as they suffer if transported. Zinnias are full-sun flowers that should be grown during the warmest parts of the summer. Be sure to water your zinnias at least once a week. For some added beauty, consider growing four o'clocks, as they bloom at night and will add a gorgeous ambiance to your gardens. Four o'clocks can be planted as early as the last frost or later into the growing season. Be sure to plant them in a permanent location and water about once a week. Four o'clocks don't experience a lot of harmful pest intervention and can encourage helpful pollinators to reside in your garden. Another flower that will attract helpful insects are cosmos flowers. Cosmos seeds should be planted directly into the soil of your raised beds at the start of summer and after there is any chance of frost. It is a great practice to sow the cosmos seeds at least a foot apart, as they rapidly expand in an enclosed area. Cosmos flowers don't need special soil requirements and can be watered semi-occasionally for the best results.

Marigolds are a particularly easy flower to grow as they don't require a lot of maintenance. Rainwater is a perfectly acceptable source of water for marigolds and you can skip watering them during your farm chores. Marigold seeds should be planted directly into your raised beds at the end of spring and early summer. They require full-sun in order to thrive. Marigolds can also act as companion plants to your vegetables because they can dissuade harmful insects from targeting your vegetables. There are three types of marigold seeds that you can buy from your local nursery: tagetes erecta, tagetes patula, and tagetes tenuifolia. Each type of marigold relates to their height and flower head size. Depending on how you want to utilize the marigolds in your garden, consider their size and structure so that you can make the most of the flower. Sunflowers are another great companion plant for vegetables. They can help beans and other vining crops that need extra vertical support. Sow the sunflower seeds directly into the soil of your raised beds. Sunflowers thrive in full-sun areas with well-draining soil that has lots of nutrients. Sunflower roots can run incredibly deep into the soil and will soak up as much as they can, so be sure to regularly add compost, mulch, and other organic fertilizers to your raised beds that have sunflowers in them. They will require semi-regular watering as they are developing.

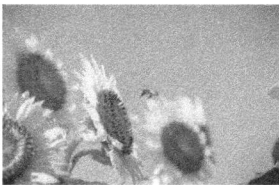

If you enjoy foraging and creating a fully edible garden, nasturtium flowers can act as a great addition. The nasturtium flower heads are fully edible and the flowers will naturally cascade. Use nasturtium flowers in raised beds for extra decorative vining flowers or in window boxes. Nasturtium flowers thrive off of rainwater alone and need very little attention to begin blossoming. The best practice for nasturtiums is to plant the seeds in their permanent location and allow them to do their thing. You can check on them occasionally if you would like, but they largely thrive when left to their own devices.

Something to keep in mind if you are planting flowers in your raised beds is that they attract slugs. A great way to get rid of slugs is to space out your flowers or add a layer of flowers at the perimeter of your garden so that they don't venture inward. You can get rid of slugs by heading out just before dawn and picking them off of your crops. *The Old Farmer's Almanac* suggests putting out a dish of beer near your garden, as this will also attract slugs and you can pick them off of the plate each morning.

9

FALL

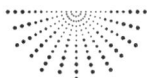

September, October, and November are the best times of the year to replant and maintain any perennial crops in your garden and start preparing for the winter. In September, remember to clean up fallen leaves. They make great additions to your compost pile but if you leave the leaves alone, they can kill your grass by smothering it and become a safety hazard because they get slimy. Be sure to collect all the leaves on your property before it rains because they become more difficult to move when they are soggy. Leaves can also be great mulch for your fruit trees. Also in September, if you have any areas on your property where you maintain a lawn, this is the best time to reseed and repair the lawn before it starts snowing. For your garden, remember to continue weeding, especially if you have perennial crops. Weeds can continue to grow throughout the fall and damage your crops.

In October, start planting spring-flowering bulbs halfway through the month and into November. You can protect your bulbs from rodents by encasing them in chicken wire. Your fruit trees and shrubs will begin their dormancy periods for the winter, be sure to avoid pruning the trees because you don't want to stimulate new growth during the winter. You can continue to plant new trees and shrubs through October so long as the ground has not frozen yet.

November is the final time that you have to prepare for the winter. There are a couple of other steps to take that I have listed at the start of the Winter section that can begin in November. As a reminder, you want to get as much done outdoors before it starts to snow. Depending on where you are in the Northeast, you may want to start these processes in October as the first snow will come early in November, or even earlier.

FALL VEGETABLES

Most of the vegetables that you have been planting so far can continue to grow through the fall. If you want to maintain some perennial crops in your garden, the fall is the best time to replant them. Some other crops to consider planting in the fall are asparagus, arugula, zucchini, shelling beans, and fennel. To start planting asparagus, dig 6 inch holes in the soil and place in the asparagus crowns. Asparagus are partial-sun plants and can be kept in shaded areas of your garden. Asparagus are perennial and can survive through the winter. In your first year, the yield of asparagus plants won't be super high but if you continue to regularly water and add compost to your asparagus, they will thrive in the following years. Arugula is a fast-growing plant that will yield harvests within a month of planting. Plant your arugula seeds consistently throughout the growing season, as they grow quickly and will begin to flower if left unattended. Once the arugula plants flower, it is time to remove them and plant new seeds. Arugula requires full sun and can be planted 3 inches apart from surrounding seeds.

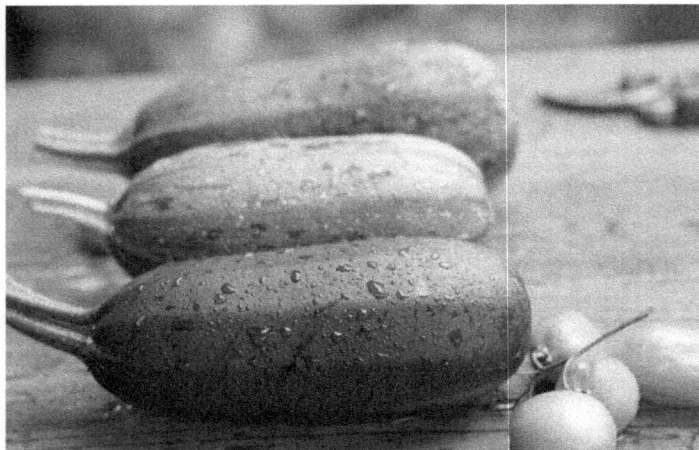

Zucchini are another easy crop to grow during your first growing season. Zucchini seeds can be planted directly into your raised bed or they can be started indoors. If you are running out of space in your raised beds and you want to practice sequential farming, start your zucchinis inside so that they are ready for transport when space opens up. Zucchinis need a spot in your garden that gets full sun and they need to be watered every week. Zucchini are very vulnerable to harmful insects, so starting them indoors will mean that you have more robust crops that can withstand a possible insect invasion. You should be ready to harvest your zucchinis when they are 6 to 8 inches long. However, if you want an extra-large zucchini, let them grow a little longer for a bigger yield.

There are two types of shelling beans that you can plant in the fall: pole beans and bush beans. Pole beans will require stakes or trellises for support. You can also utilize companion planting and plant pole beans near sunflowers or corn so that they can use the strong and tall plants for support. You can expect the first harvest of your beans 6 weeks after planting them. Bush beans are shorter plants that make a great addition to raised beds because they don't need a lot of space to grow. You can expect your first harvest of bush beans 3 to 4 weeks after they are planted. Both types of beans can be directly planted into the soil of your garden and don't need to be started indoors. Shelling beans are full-sun crops that require minimal water and can thrive on rain-water alone. Be sure to harvest all of your beans quickly to maximize your yields during the fall.

There are two types of fennel that you can grow in your fall garden: Florence fennel and sweet fennel. Florence fennel is an annual crop that will need to be replanted each year. Sweet fennel is perennial and can survive relatively mild winters outdoors, or you can transport them into your greenhouse at the end of the season to preserve them for the following year. Both types of fennel are full-sun crops that require weekly watering. Fennel will attract both helpful and harmful insects to your garden. If you are seeing small green caterpillars attracted to your fennel, consider planting Queen Anne's lace nearby and transporting the caterpillars to the flower. Carrot rust flies are also attracted to fennel and they can damage the crop. Consider covering your outdoor fennel with a mesh fabric to keep the flies away.

FALL FRUITS AND HERBS

Again, you can continue to plant new fruit trees and berry bushes through the fall months but be sure not to prune them as they are getting ready for the winter. You can add grapes, cranberries, and chicory to the list of fruits and herbs that are growing in your garden. Any herbs that you have in your garden that you want to continue enjoying throughout the winter need to be repotted and moved indoors or into your greenhouse during the fall. Grapes can be started in May or June once the last frost has cleared your area. However, many fruit trees and shrubs are best planted in the fall so that they have time to develop a deep root system. There are many different varieties of grapevines that you can choose from when you are starting grapes on your farm. The difference in variety indicates what you will do with them. If you are growing grapes to make wine, consider growing Frontenac, La Crescent, Marquette, Swenson white, or St. Croix grapes. If you are growing grapes to eat or to make into jelly, consider growing Bluebell, Edelweiss, or Swenson red grapes. The seedless grape varieties that you can grow in the northeast are Mars, Petite Jewel, and Somerset Seedless. To plant your grapevines, soak the vines in water for a couple of hours before you plant them. Grapevines don't need to be planted too deep into the soil but will require initial supports from stakes or trellises. Watering your grapevines can mostly be accomplished from rainwater in the early weeks of growth. If you are going through a heat wave or drought, be sure to water your grapes at least once a week.

There are two types of cranberries that you can grow on your Northeast farm: North American cranberries and North American low-bush cranberries. The North American cranberries are the classic Thanksgiving cranberries that are tart and best eaten with sugar. The North American low-bush cranberries act just like other fruit shrubs and can be eaten directly off the vine. While most classic cranberries are grown in bogs, this is not necessary for growing great cranberries on your farm. Both types of cranberries require moist soil. When you are planting your cranberries, dig an area that is 10 inches deep into the soil and plant your cranberries 2 feet apart. Fill the 10-inch hole with peat moss and fertilizer for the best results. Cranberries are a long-term investment and you won't actually see any fruit until they are 3 years old. However, both types of cranberries are delicious and can add a lot of value to your farm. They may require some protection during the winter but don't worry, they are cold-hardy and will survive the Northeast winters.

Chicory seeds are started indoors typically 5 weeks before they are transplanted outdoors. Chicory will grow best if transported in the early weeks of September. Sow the seeds 6 inches into the soil and 2 feet apart from surrounding crops. Chicory will thrive if temperatures remain below 75 °F, which makes them perfect fall crops. Be sure to water your chicory at least once a week and transport the plant back indoors or to your greenhouse before the winter.

FALL FLOWERS

The work that you will be doing with the flowers in your garden during the fall is mostly going to consist of prep for the winter and following spring. Many of the bulb flowers that you have in your garden at this point will have made daughter bulbs that you can dig up and replant. Additionally, you can add wildflowers and Persian buttercups to your fall gardens for the last bits of color for the year. Wildflowers are a great project to get started in the fall, as they require very minimal maintenance and can attract helpful insects to your gardens. Wildflowers are native to different areas in the Northeast; be sure to get a mix of wildflower seeds that are native to your area so as to not introduce invasive species to your garden. Planting wildflowers in the fall will mean that they will remain dormant during the winter and blossom in the spring. Wildflower seeds are a great option for the perimeter of your raised beds or to add color to an area of your property that is lacking it. When you till the soil for your wildflower seeds, be sure the seeds are planted 1 to 2 inches into the soil. For the first few weeks after planting your wildflowers, be sure to water the area at least once a week so that the seeds can properly germinate. Once the flowers are 1 to 2 inches tall, you can stop watering and let the rainwater handle your wildflowers. If you are finding that your wildflowers are looking dull, you can mow the area with a tall mower or weed whacker. Persian buttercups are annual flowers in the Northeast that can be planted in either the spring or fall. When you are planting your Persian buttercups in the fall, be sure to transport them back indoors for the winter. When planting the buttercup tubers, you will need to plant them 2 inches deep into the soil and 6 inches apart. They are full-sun flowers that require bi-weekly watering.

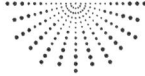

There are a couple more seasonal chores that need to be completed at the start of the winter season on your farm. Depending on where you are in the Northeast, these chores may need to be started in late October and can run through the beginning of December. First, ensure that any outdoor water sources are drained and stored for the winter months. Be sure to shut off any water valves that are exposed to the elements so that they do not freeze, which can cause burst pipes. Cover the faucets for winter with protective coverings so that they don't leak or freeze. Next, take another walk through your property and note any damage that you need to repair for the winter. Cracks, scratches, and holes in your existing struc-

tures can lead to intense drafts in the winter that
will suck away all your warm air. Last, shelter your
raised beds. In December or earlier (definitely before
the first snow), be sure to cover your perennial crops
with mulch and turn the soil. If you have perennial
crops growing in your raised beds, be sure to cover
them with their preferred coverings. If you are
transporting crops back indoors or to your greenhouse, now is the time to do so.

December is also a great
time to get hardwood
cuttings from your trees and
shrubs. These hardwood
cuttings can be sprinkled
over your raised beds to protect them from the frost
and decompose for a more robust soil in the spring.
Some of the trees and shrubs that you may plant in
December could have bagworms; be sure to remove
these by hand. This is also your last chance to
inspect the fencing around your property for holes
or tears before the snow comes in full force. As an
additional deterrent to any deer or other wild
animals, hang a bar of soap in cheese cloth from a
tree near the perimeter of your property. Animals
don't like the smell as it reminds them of humans
and they will stay away.

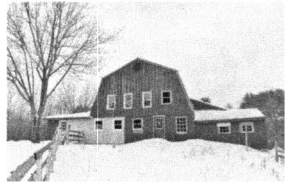

The winter season on your Northeast farm doesn't have to just be a barren expanse of land. Winter can bring color, vibrancy, and new opportunities, just like any other season. While you may not be able to tend to your garden as much as you may have grown accustomed to, you can spend your time observing your farm and looking at new areas for improvement. During the winter, after all of the leaves have fallen, you have the opportunity to see where you have gaps on your property. It may be that you have a lot of space that was once covered by tree branches, to add a new structure or expand your garden. Take the winter to plan out and research new ideas for your homestead and practice the permaculture principle of observation.

Winter is also a great time to consider your view. When the trees no longer have their leaves, you can see much more clearly across your farm. It may be the case that your neighbors now have direct sight onto your property. Consider where you'd like to plant new trees and shrubs in the following seasons. You can also spend the time manicuring your property, provided that the temperature doesn't deter you from going outside. If you get that itch to be active in nature, you can do some needed clean up on your property. I am sure at this point in the year you have overgrown trees or bushes that are merely part of the landscape. Take the time to trim them down and create a more cohesive looking farm.

WINTER TREES AND SHRUBS

While these are some ideas for how to spend your winter, there are certainly more options for gardening to consider this season. You don't have to spend your winter staring at a blank gray and white scene. Instead, consider planting cold-hardy winter trees and shrubs. The winter trees that thrive in the Northeast are juniper trees, evergreens, euonymus, and nandina trees. Red twig dogwood, cherry laurels, and winterberry holly shrubs can also add a pop of color to your farm.

There are many different varieties of juniper trees and bushes and you can choose from many different winter-hardy varieties for your farm. When you are planting juniper trees, be sure to find a spot that gets at least 6 hours of sun per day. Dig a small trench around the base of your juniper trees so that the soil can drain from snow or rain. Other than that, junipers are very easy to grow and will add vibrancy to your winter farm. If you are thinking about adding evergreen trees to your property, consider purchasing saplings rather than trying to propagate the trees on your own. Propagation of trees is a tricky process that may require additional research to do correctly for your area. Planting evergreen saplings is a great place to start and can add a bit of holiday cheer to your property. Most evergreen trees want access to the sun, so find a spot on your farm that gets direct sun for a lot of the day. When you find the right spot, dig up a hole for the base of the tree to rest in. You want the soil to be looser than the surrounding area so that the evergreen tree roots can take hold. Water the soil and roots considerably when you first plant the tree so that the roots are well hydrated. If you are planting your trees at the end of fall or beginning of winter, be sure to add a trench around the base of the tree so that any precipitation can drain through the soil.

Euonymus plants can be another addition to your winter farm. They tolerate any type of sun or shade condition and are incredibly resilient. There are six types of euonymus plants that you can add to your farm: wintercreeper, evergreen, America, winged, spindle, and spreading euonymus. Be sure to plant euonymus before the first snow because they do well when planted in dry conditions. Nandinas are another great option for your winter farm that will speckle your landscape with a gorgeous red color in the winter. They are not picky about the amount of sun that they get, so add them wherever you want on your farm. Nandina do require good soil drainage in the early weeks of their growing cycle. Be sure to add a trench around the plant to support better drainage. You will want to buy nandina saplings from a nursery and gently loosen their roots before planting.

Red twig dogwood is a great shrub to add to your winter landscape that is not picky and very resilient. Like the nandina, you can plant the red twig dogwood in full sun or full shade and it will thrive. This shrub is a fast grower and will require some light pruning during the winter, but the added pop of red to your farm is definitely worth it. Winterberry holly can also add some seasonal color to your winter farm and produce adorable berries in the summer, but don't eat them; they are merely there for aesthetic purposes. The holly bushes do best in full sun or partial shade. Be sure to fully saturate the soil before planting the holly bushes because they do best in moist soil. There are eight varieties of winterberry holly that you can choose from that are native to the Northeast: Aurantiaca, Berry Poppins,

Cacapon, La Have, Oosterwijk, Red Sprite, Winter Red, and Winter Gold.

The best time to plant cherry laurels is in the late fall and early winter. They are cold-hardy plants that will blossom in the spring. They too need a sunny area with well-draining soil in order to thrive. Water the cherry laurel for the first few weeks and then allow the roots to take hold during the winter. In the spring, add fresh fertilizer and compost to the soil around the cherry laurel for the best results.

TIPS AND TRICKS FOR ULTIMATE SUCCESS

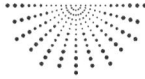

iguring out your homestead design is an essential step when you are starting on a new property. In Chapter 6, I covered permaculture design principles and the ways to incorporate those principles on to your farm. Now I want to discuss some more tips and tricks to keep in mind when you are beginning a new farm. The first tip is to discover your short-term and long-term goals. This is a great way to inform the design of your farm. If you have a short-term goal or raising ducks, then you need to decide how and where to build a duck coop, a water source for them, and ways to automate their feeding times. If you have a long-term goal of setting up a home orchard, then you might section off a piece of land and reserve the area for your orchard when you are ready to tackle the project.

Next, make a list of the large-scale projects that you may want to accomplish. I discussed this briefly in an earlier section. I can't stress the importance of designing from the idea down to the small details. When you are deciding which large-scale projects you want to accomplish on your farm you need to do a lot of research to develop how you are going to tackle the projects. If you are building a greenhouse, how are you going to build it, what materials will you need, and will you require contract work to accomplish the project? Ask yourself these questions and then detail the exact expenses for every aspect. This practice has the added benefit of giving you an eye for details. Once you get in the habit of detailing every minute detail of a project, you will start doing this on your farm and in your home. Considering the small details and ensuring that everything is working with a purpose is crucial to a self-sustaining lifestyle. It will also mean that you aren't spending frivolous money on projects that could have been accomplished if more details were fleshed out.

While I have written at length about the importance of planning and observing your property before you start building or farming, you need to also consult your city or county. Every region has specific zoning laws that need to be adhered to. You may also be in an area with a Homeowners Association that has regulations about what you can and cannot do on your property. Be sure to consult the regulations and laws for your area so that you don't invest time and resources into a project just to find out that you can't have it. When I knew that I wanted to start homesteading, I started a small garden in my backyard and put up some trellises to practice some farming techniques. I found out after a few weeks that the location of my garden violated the Homeowners Association's regulations for my area. I had to completely dismantle the garden and relocate all of my crops. I ended up losing a lot of my plants in the process. Don't be like me: do the research first so that you don't have to tear down a project that you worked hard on.

Something that I think a lot of people overlook on their first property is fencing. Fences, whether man-made or organic, should be some of the first expenses for your property. Fencing can help, especially in the Northeast, to keep deer and other larger animals off of your property. It also has the added benefit of keeping any small critters or children safely *on* your property. Raised beds also count as fencing against smaller rodents that may have found their way onto your land. These initial investments are critical to the long-term success of your farm.

OPTIMIZING THE SPACE ON YOUR PROPERTY

An area of your home that I cannot stress the importance of enough is storage. Whether you invest in a survival storage system or just an everyday storage system, storage will be key to keeping your house chaos-free and streamlining some of your processes. You want to have access to quality storage on your farm so that you can preserve your produce and ensure that your family always has food. In the Northeast, you are bound to get long and cold winters, where your capacity for gardening will be limited. Ensuring that you have a substantial storage system to keep all of your goods fresh will make the winters seem like a breeze. My biggest tip for storage is to set this up before you start working outside on your property. You are going to want to have plenty of shelving, a couple of refrigerators, and some freezers to preserve the harvest from your garden.

PLANTING SUCCESS

Planting for successful growing seasons requires a lot of attention to detail and a plan for how you are going to create environments for your diverse garden to thrive. I suggest starting your own planting calendar. *The Old Farmer's Almanac* has a general planting calendar on their website that lists the best times to start plants indoors and outdoors throughout the growing season. In the Northeast, due to the varied temperatures, I suggest creating your own. A planting calendar will be able to tell you what dates you should start seeds, depending on the first and last frosts of the year. This style of planning will maximize your yields. Starting plants indoors will mean that they will be ready to harvest quicker once you transport them outdoors. A planting calendar can also account for rain. If you create your own planting calendar you can add a tracking system for rain days. Knowing when it has rained will also influence how often you need to water specific plants, as well as the best time to plant new crops. Another benefit of planting calendars is that they are uniquely useful if you are using a sequential farming method. Sequentially farming different crops using a planting calendar can help you map out when to rotate out a crop after it has been harvested so that you have a bountiful garden all year long.

In addition to a planting calendar, I also want to encourage you to learn how to propagate new plants from clippings. Propagation is a money-saving farming technique that allows you to start new crops from the clippings of existing plants in your garden. This is also great if you love a particular crop and want to continue growing it in your greenhouse over the winter months. Propagation is safe for plants and can save you a lot of money in the first couple of years on your farm. Why spend extra money on plants at the nursery if you can take a clipping from your garden and grow an entirely new plant?

Water sources are another consideration that will be crucial in the beginning phases of planning your property. Collect rainwater in bins for your gardens. Rainwater is gentle and incredibly rich in nutrients. There are other irrigation systems that you can implement once you expand your gardening opera-tion. However, in the beginning, invest in some rain-water collection bins and reroute that water to your gardens. Another DIY-friendly watering method is to collect your wine and other glass bottles to use as drip irrigators. Placing water in a wine bottle and sticking the nose of the wine bottle into the soil will allow the water to slowly drain in the soil. If you have followed the previously mentioned steps about how to have quality soil with good drainage, drip irrigators are a great option. The water will slowly drain through the soil and the root system of nearby crops will absorb the water. You can even use recycled soda bottles as drip irrigators and there is more flexibility with the style and breadth of irrigation with plastic bottles.

The last water management tip that I want to tell you about is a *greywater* system. Greywater systems have become incredibly popular as more people are moving in tiny homes and vans. Greywater is the water that you have used in your kitchen, shower, or sinks. You can collect this water and reuse it for other purposes around your farm. Utilizing the greywater on your farm is a sustainable practice that is healthy and eco-friendly. Greywater systems are also energy efficient because instead of pumping water into the sewer or septic tank, you can reroute the water to your garden.

INSECT MANAGEMENT

I have briefly mentioned the benefits of helpful insects in your garden and ways to avoid harmful insects. However, there are some more concrete ways to improve your garden by decreasing the harmful insect population and increasing the helpful population. The first and most important step is to ensure that you have clean and quality soil. If you start with soil that is uninhabitable to your crops, you will attract harmful insects and diseases to your garden. Clean soil is soil that is rich in helpful organic matter and has been layered and tilled with compost and mulch. Refer back to Chapter 5 for a more in-depth look at how to treat your soil.

Once you have established clean soil, you will want to water your crops in the morning, control weeds and regularly clean out your gardens, and aggressively thin out your plants. Watering your plants in the morning allows your plants to perform photosynthesis during the day and dry off by the time night falls. It is also more efficient as the heat of the sun often evaporates water before it reaches the plants if you water during the day. If your plants are damp during the colder parts of the day, they can become overridden with mold and attract harmful insects. If you are not an early riser, drip irrigators and soakers are a great investment to make so that your plants are watered in the morning while you are still sleeping.

Controlling the weeds in your garden will also decrease harmful pest intervention and allow your plants to thrive. Weeds compete with your plants for space and nutrients and are notoriously aggressive growers. Using the permaculture methods and companion planting in your raised beds will eliminate a lot of the space that weeds could take up. It is a generally great practice to weed your garden every week or every other week as you continue to work on your farm. This goes hand in hand with ensuring that your garden is clean. Remove fallen leaves and twigs from your garden as they can introduce new harmful insects. You can also improve the rate of decomposition in your compost by regularly adding the debris that you find in your garden to the compost pile. Accomplish two tasks at once by keeping your garden clean: aggressively thinning plants is a way to avoid weaker plants that are prone to diseases from spreading those diseases to other plants; and thinning plants can also remove harmful insect larvae and eggs from your garden. Prune dead leaves, shoots, and branches from your garden so that you can restore airflow to struggling plants.

You will also want to promote helpful insect populations in your garden. A great way to do this is to add some pollinating flowers to your garden to attract bees and butterflies. If you are raising chickens, you can also allow your chickens to roam through your garden for controlled periods of time, as they will eat a lot of the harmful insects that are hiding among the plants. Similarly, ladybugs, praying mantises, and wasps are other beneficial garden insects that you can entice to your garden with their preferred flowers. If you are buying helpful insects to introduce to your garden, avoid any chemical insecticides. Chemicals in your garden will kill any insects that reside there, regardless of their usefulness to your garden. The last way to promote a healthy garden with helpful insects is to rotate your crops. I wrote briefly about this in Chapter 6, but rotating your crops can reduce the risk of plant disease and will mean that harmful insects have a harder time locating specific crops on which to feed.

Leave a 1-Click Review!

Customer reviews

⭐⭐⭐⭐⭐ 5 out of 5

3 global ratings

5 star		100%
4 star		0%
3 star		0%
2 star		0%
1 star		0%

⌄ How are ratings calculated?

Review this product

Share your thoughts with other customers

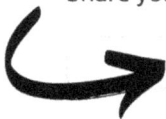

Write a customer review

AFTERWORD

Starting a homestead in the Northeast is an excellent opportunity to cultivate a farm that experiences all four seasons, engage in a sustainable lifestyle, and bring an overall happiness to your life that you might be missing. The essential tools that you will need when you are starting your Northeast farm are to take your time and do as much research as you can. This is your journey and finding the best ways to do things doesn't need to be a rushed process. Consider the permaculture design principles when you start designing your homestead. Remember to center the projects that you want to accomplish on your farm with an adherence to the natural flow of the ecological systems around you. Homesteading and permaculture protocols and principles will not only help save the planet, they will also streamline everything for you in a very productive fashion.

In the Northeast, the seasonal changes demand a lot of attention. The benefits of these changes are that you can get a wider range of plants in your garden and you can learn more about horticultural principles for each plant. Becoming a master at your craft will take time and on a Northeast farm: you have so much more access to different plants and methods than in other areas. Take your time while you are engaging with these practices. For the most success on your farm, don't do anything major during the first year on your property. Take some time to just observe the land and establish ideas for projects that you may want to implement.

Overall, the homesteading journey is one that will span many years. Many people who start homestead farms call their properties their 'forever homes.' Finding your forever home means that you have plenty of time to spare. Not only will living in tandem with nature fuel your happiness, but it will make you a healthier person at the same time. Sustainability means working with what you have and if you have a vegetable garden on your farm, then you will definitely be eating more greens and less processed foods.

When you put down this book, I want you to consider all of the projects that you have bubbling up in your mind. Write down as many as you can and keep them around. Then, once you get onto your property, really observe what is around you. Learn to roll with the changes that you will face as a result of learning how to live on your property. The worst thing you can do is try and force a project into place when the ecology around you is fighting the project. Creating the tangible first steps for your homestead is a great way to begin because you are engaging your mind and thinking critically about the nature around you.

At the end of the day, this is your journey and the pace that you set for your journey is completely your own. Remember to stay focused on the overarching goal that homesteading is a long-term project and investment. There will be setbacks and obstacles to overcome, but mastering your craft and learning new lessons will make them a more pleasurable experience. If you are considering the homesteading lifestyle and you want to be part of a community of people who are doing the same, join our Facebook group: Northeast Homestead Gardeners and Foragers. In this group we discuss more detailed tips and tricks about starting your Northeast farm.

There are also community members who will be willing to give you direct feedback about your farm that is tailored to your experience. If you found this book helpful for your homesteading journey, consider leaving a review to help other people learn skills for their first farm. I wish you all the luck in the world as you start your journey into farming in the Northeast!

Other Titles!

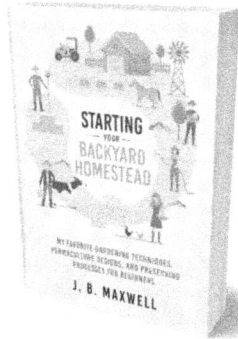

https://www.amazon.com/dp/B09PK252MF

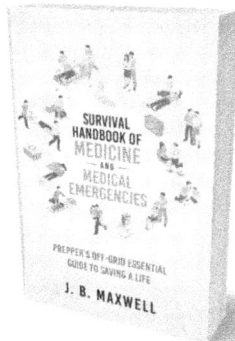

Survival Handbook of
Medicine and Medical
Emergencies (coming soon)

REFERENCES

A prescription for better health: Go alfresco. (2010, October 12). Harvard Health. https://www.health.harvard.edu/mind-and-mood/a-prescription-for-better-health-go-alfresco

Ananda. (2021, February 1). *28 best DIY raised bed garden ideas & designs.* A Piece of Rainbow. https://www.apieceofrainbow.com/20-diy-raised-bed-gardens/

April. (2016, June 2). *Getting into the permaculture zone.* Permaculture Visions. https://permaculturevisions.com/getting-permaculture-zone/

Autumn. (2017, March 6). *10 principles to live by for homesteading newbies.* A Traditional Life. https://atraditionallife.com/10-things-you-should-know-about-homesteading/

Berg Stack, L. (2017). *Soil and plant nutrition: A gardener's perspective*. Cooperative Extension: Garden & Yard; The University of Maine. https://extension.umaine.edu/gardening/manual/soils/soil-and-plant-nutrition/

BigRentz Inc. (2020, April 7). *How to build a life off the grid*. BigRentz. https://www.bigrentz.com/blog/off-grid-living

Bloom, J. (2016, August 2). *The basics of permaculture*. Mother Earth Living. https://content.motherearthliving.com/gardening/basics-of-permaculture-zmgz16sozolc/

Carlson, S. (2018, April 18). *What's the best type of soil for plants?* Peterson Companies. https://blog.petersoncompanies.net/best-type-of-soil-for-plants

Cowan, S. (2019, March 26). *10 expert tips for raised garden beds and planters*. Eartheasy Guides & Articles. https://learn.eartheasy.com/articles/10-expert-tips-for-raised-garden-beds-and-planters/

Culver, B. (2021, May 19). *What is homesteading?* An off Grid Life. https://www.anoffgridlife.com/what-is-homesteading/

Faires, N. (2017). *10 excellent reasons to use raised beds in your garden*. Eartheasy Guides & Articles. https://learn.eartheasy.com/articles/10-excellent-reasons-to-use-raised-beds-in-your-garden/

Family Food Garden. (2018, December 10). *Design your homestead & backyard farm plans.* Family Food Garden. https://www.familyfoodgarden.com/homestead-backyard-farm/

Garden Heights Nursery. (2018, April 2). *What's the difference between perennial and annual plants?* Garden Heights Nursery. https://www.garden-heights.com/single-post/2018/03/30/whats-the-difference-between-perennial-and-annual-plants#:~:text=So%2C%20what%27s%20the%20difference%3F

Garman, J. (2017, January 20). *The basics of raising chickens.* Homesteaders of America. https://homesteadersofamerica.com/basics-raising-chickens/

Homesteading Family. (2020, September 6). *The first 7 things you must do on your new homestead property.* [Video] https://www.youtube.com/watch?v=sZ5wJc7v7Qs&ab_channel=HomesteadingFamily

Kellogg Garden Products. (2021). *Benefits of companion planting.* Kellogg Garden. https://www.kellogggarden.com/blog/gardening/benefits-of-companion-planting/

Lynn, T. (2020, March 18). *10 wonderful benefits of chickens.* Simple Living Country Gal. https://simplelivingcountrygal.com/benefits-of-chickens

Martin, S. (n.d.). *10 essential spring gardening tasks.*

Proven Winners. https://www.provenwinners.com/learn/early-spring/10-essential-spring-gardening-tasks

Melanie. (2020, August 1). *How much does it cost to start beekeeping? (Updated 2021)*. Beekeeping For Newbies. https://www.beekeepingfo rnewbies.com/starting-costs/

Milbrand, L. (2021, September 29). *A beginner's guide to indoor composting (without worms!)*. Real Simple. https://www.realsimple.com/home-organizing/green-living/indoor-composting

National Climate Assessment. (2021). *Northeast*. National Climate Assessment. https://nca2014.globalchange.gov/report/regions/northeast

Page, T. (2016, December 9). *Homestead goats: What you need to know to get started*. Common Sense Home. https://commonsensehome.com/homestead-goats/

Patterson, S. (n.d.). *Which soil is best for plant growth?* LoveToKnow. https://garden.lovetoknow.com/wiki/Which_Soil_Is_Best_for_Plant_Growth

RIMOL Greenhouse Systems. (2018, September 19). *How to achieve ideal environmental control in your greenhouse*. Rimol Greenhouses. https://www.rimol-greenhouses.com/blog/how-to-achieve-ideal-environmental-control-your-greenhouse

Sayner, A. (2021, July 20). *17 backyard homestead ideas for living independently.* GroCycle. https://grocycle.com/backyard-homestead-ideas/

Tilley, N. (2018, January 12). *What is a permaculture garden: The essence of permaculture gardening.* Gardening Know How. https://www.gardeningknowhow.com/special/organic/the-essence-of-permaculture-gardening.htm

Tropical Permaculture. (n.d.). *What is permaculture? How does permaculture work? Explanations, definitions, examples.* Tropical Permaculture. https://www.tropicalpermaculture.com/what-is-permaculture.html

US EPA. (2016, December). *Climate impacts in the Northeast.* Environmental Protection Agency. https://19january2017snapshot.epa.gov/climate-impacts/climate-impacts-northeast_.html

Vanderlinden, C. (2021, January 4). *10 tips for successful raised-bed gardening.* The Spruce. https://www.thespruce.com/tips-for-successful-raised-bed-gardening-2539792

Vanheems, B. (2019, January 11). *10 ways to boost yields in your vegetable garden.* GrowVeg. https://www.growveg.com/guides/10-ways-to-boost-yields-in-your-vegetable-garden/

Vinje, E. (2012, December 8). *Companion planting*

guide. Planet Natural. https://www.planetnatural.-com/companion-planting/

Watson, M. (2019, September 27). *What's in season? A monthly guide to the Northeast's fruits and veggies*. The Spruce Eats. https://www.thespruceeats.com/seasonal-fruits-and-vegetables-of-the-north-east-4165314

WeatherSpark. (2020). *Climate and average weather year round in North East*. Weatherspark. https://weatherspark.com/y/22771/Average-Weather-in-North-East-Maryland-United-States-Year-Round#: ~:text=

In%20North%20East%2C%20the%20summers

Winger, J. (2014, May 14). *Become a beekeeper: 8 steps to getting started with honeybees*. The Prairie Homestead. https://www.theprairiehomestead.-com/2014/05/get-started-honeybees.html

All photos sourced from Unsplash. https://unsplash.com/

www.ingramcontent.com/pod-product-compliance
Lightning Source LLC
Chambersburg PA
CBHW032057020426
42335CB00011B/380